‖‖‖ ‖‖ ‖‖‖‖ ‖‖‖‖‖‖‖‖‖‖‖‖‖‖‖‖ ‖‖‖‖‖‖‖ ‖ ‖‖ ‖‖‖

KT-116-209

Everything you ever wanted to ask about

Royal Borough of Windsor and Maidenhead	
214863	
PETERS	31-Mar-06
612.6	

Tricia Kreitman, Dr Neil Simpson
& Dr Rosemary Jones

Illustrated by Kathryn Lamb

Piccadilly Press • London

*We would like to dedicate this book to all the men in
our lives (and the women in Neil's)*

RBWM LIBRARY SERVICES			
MMAI		METO	
MWIN		METW	
MASC		MOLD	
MCOO		MSUN	
MDAT		MCON	
MDED			

First published in Great Britain in 2002
by Piccadilly Press Ltd.

Text copyright © Tricia Kreitman, Neil Simpson
and Rosemary Jones, 2002
Illustrations © Kathryn Lamb, 2002

All rights reserved. No part of this publication may be reproduced,
stored in a retrieval system, or transmitted in any form or by any
means, electronic, mechanical, photocopying, recording or
otherwise, without the prior permission of the copyright owner.

The right of Tricia Kreitman, Neil Simpson and Rosemary Jones,
to be identified as Authors of this work has been asserted by them
in accordance with the Copyright, Designs and Patents Act 1988

A catalogue record for this book is available from the British Library

ISBN: 1 85340 634 1 (trade paperback)
1 85340 639 2 (hardback)

5 7 9 10 8 6 4

Printed and bound in Great Britain by Bookmarque Ltd.
Design by Judith Robertson
Cover design by Fielding Design

Set in 10.5/16pt Futura Book

Contents

Acknowledgements

We would like to thank all the boys and young men who helped us with this book by talking to us, confiding their problems, answering our questions and telling us what they really wanted to know. We are particularly grateful to Geoff, Ed and his friends, Richard and his friends, Mark Dexter and the young men at HMYOI Lancaster Farms, Viv Crouch and her pupils, and Jane Dale and the boys at The Priory LSST.

How to Use This Book

- ◇ Everything in this book is based on what real boys have said they really want to know.
- ◇ You may choose to read straight through from the beginning to the end, or just pick out the sections that sound most interesting to you.
- ◇ Apart from Chapter 1, each chapter begins with a list of the topics covered in that section.
- ◇ Most chapters also have true-life stories and/or problem pages.
- ◇ Finally, because it's so hard to talk about your body and what's happening inside you without using some medical or technical names, we've made a list (glossary) with words you might not know. You can find this at the back of the book.

Introduction

At school we got the lesson about boys and girls being different and how you had to treat each other well and all that – and then, about three years later they started talking about teenage pregnancy. There was nothing in between; you just had to go through puberty on your own. The trouble was, by the time they started talking to you about sex and birth control, you were already a ticking testosterone time bomb! Geoff, 25

For 16 years I have worked as an agony aunt for a teenage magazine. Every week, along with sackloads of mail from girls and young women, there were a few letters from boys. Some asked for very simple, basic information. Others had more complicated problems or were worried about a friend or family member. The girls who wrote would often have discussed their problem first with friends or family, but the boys frequently said they were too embarrassed to ask for help or admit their ignorance.

The questions boys ask include:

◇ *When will I start to get taller?*
◇ *How can I control my squeaky voice?*
◇ *When will my private parts start to get bigger?*
◇ *How large should my penis be?*

◇ *Should I worry about spots on my penis?*
◇ *Does everyone think about suicide sometimes?*
◇ *Do girls think about sex as much as boys?*

For the past six years I have been working with a group of consultant paediatricians (doctors specialising in children's and young people's medicine). They work with young people in schools and clinics and had been hearing the same types of questions. We started looking more closely at the situation and realised several things:

◇ Lessons in school about puberty and growing up often tell boys (and girls) too little, too late.
◇ Many parents find it difficult or even impossible to talk about sexual development with their sons.
◇ The information that parents or schools do give is often biological rather than practical.

Boys do very often prefer to ask factual questions, but this doesn't mean they don't also suffer from emotional concerns and problems. Unfortunately, sex education – particularly for boys – often centres on what you do rather than how you feel. We asked hundreds of boys and young men how puberty felt for them. They told us what they really wanted to know – or what they would have liked to know when it was happening to them.

This book isn't written for professionals and parents – although they may be interested to see what's in it! Instead, we wrote it especially for boys who are going through puberty and sexual development. I hope this will give them the answers to some of their worries, or at least the confidence to ask for more help and advice if they need it.

Tricia Kreitman

Chapter 1

Why Do I Need to Know All This?

This book is about growing up and the changes that happen to your body – particularly your penis and the other bits which develop as you become a man. All these changes are normal, so you might wonder what the fuss is about! We decided to write this guide to willies and boys' bits because so many boys and young men had asked us for advice and information. You might also find it useful for the following reasons:

◇ **Because it's something everyone goes through.** The growing up process – or puberty – starts at different times for different people. Even if you haven't yet noticed any changes in yourself, it will happen – probably soon. Once puberty starts, changes can happen quickly. It makes sense to find out as much as possible so you're really well prepared.

◇ **Because many people (parents included) find it difficult to talk openly to boys about their bodies.** It's often easier to make a joke about willies than to openly discuss the kind of problems you can get with your penis. For many people it's an embarrassing or even a taboo subject. Many grown-ups wouldn't know how to ask for help themselves, never mind give you advice. It's not surprising that people grow up feeling it's wrong to talk about their bodies – and that any worries should be suffered in silence.

◇ **Because, although you probably have lessons about puberty and growing up in school, these may concentrate more on biology than practical advice.** Understanding what's going on inside your body is very important, but many boys have worries about whether their willies are normal, how they should cope with their changing emotions, or even about negotiating with their parents for more privacy and respect now that they're growing up. It's these practical but important questions that are often left unanswered in school biology and sex education lessons.

◇ **Because you might hear myths and rumours, and it's important to know the truth.** Because bodies and sex are still such embarrassing topics for so many people, there are lots of misunderstandings around. For example, you might hear that masturbation is bad or dangerous or be worried that your penis seems crooked and points to the right or the left. In fact masturbation is a normal part of growing up and getting to know your own body. Obviously it's something you would only want to do in private, but it won't harm

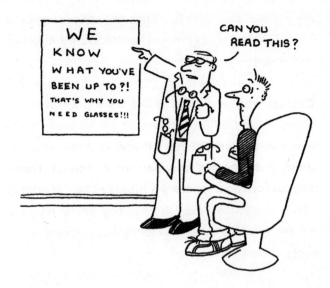

you. It relieves some of the sexual tension built up by all those hormones rushing around in your blood, and it's an excellent way of finding out what feels good for you. And lots of willies look slightly bent on erection. Unless it's causing you pain or other problems there's no need to worry. Once you learn more about boys' bodies and how they work and read the problem pages in this book you'll be able to sort out fact from fiction.

◇ **Because although growing up is normal, it's also normal to have worries or questions.** When your body begins to change, your voice breaks and you get hair on your face and other places, it's only natural to have some questions. Things can happen that you may not be too sure about or would like some

15

advice on. Hopefully this book will answer a lot of these questions – or give you the confidence to ask for further help if you need it.

⬦ **Because so many boys suffer from peer pressure about their bodies, it's important to understand that everyone is different.** People start puberty at different times and, even then, some grow quickly and others more slowly. Many boys feel worried and left out because their bodies are 'different' in some way. Knowing that it's OK not to be the same as your friends can help you to stop worrying.

⬦ **Because your friends might not be as clued up as you, and you can help them out.**

OK, so lots of boys don't like talking about personal problems, but you aren't the only one these things are happening to. Some of your friends are going to have their own fears and worries. Once you've read this book you'll be in a very good position to help them cope, because you'll know the answers to those difficult questions that nobody else seems quite sure about.

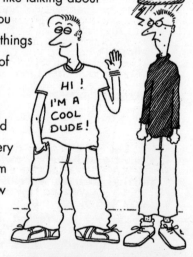

... SOME GROW QUICKLY AND OTHERS MORE SLOWLY.

◇ **Because the media will be firing images and advertising at you and playing on your fears about your body.** Look at the messages underneath many ads and you'll see they're playing on people's insecurities. Would you be more successful with girls if you drank this beer, used this shampoo or covered yourself in this deodorant? Advertisers know that if they can get you using their product while you're still quite young, there's a chance you'll stay loyal to it for a long time. So they're going to spend a lot of money to persuade you that theirs is not only best, but also essential for you. For example, many spot creams and lotions are excellent, but for some people they're just not strong enough. You could spend a fortune in response to the advertising and still suffer from acne. What you really need is to ask the pharmacist for something stronger or talk to your doctor about prescription medication. Understanding the different options can help you see through some of the advertising hype and make decisions for yourself.

And . . .

◇ **Because thousands of boys have told us that these are the things they really wanted to know.**

Chapter 2

Puberty: What the Outside World Sees

This chapter covers:
- ◇ The meaning of puberty
- ◇ When it's likely to happen
- ◇ How your body changes
- ◇ What causes it
- ◇ Body size and shape
- ◇ Body hair
- ◇ Spots and smells
- ◇ Voice breaking
- ◇ Delayed puberty

A boy's body changes from something like this . . .

This chapter explains the changes that other people will notice as you grow and go through puberty. You may already know some – or even a lot – of this from school or other books.

What Does Puberty Mean?

Puberty is the word that describes all the changes that take place as you grow from being a child into an adult.

Your first sign of puberty might be some new body hair or an awareness that your testes are growing larger. The

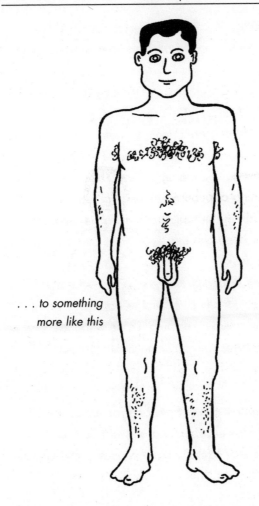

. . . to something more like this

process ends when you're a fully grown man; much taller with a different body shape. On the way your voice will deepen (or break) and your penis will grow larger and start to behave as though it has a mind of its own! More about some of these more personal changes in Chapter 3.

I think I was about 12 when I started to notice that my body was changing. I grew taller and began to get hair on my face, etc.

Nico, 19

Hair was the first thing – it suddenly starts growing in certain places like chest and legs. It's quite a trophy at the beginning and you can compare yourself to other people and feel good. Hair is certainly taken to be a sign of growing up and people comment on your hairiness. It's embarrassing but inside you're secretly quite pleased.

Sam, 17

I was 12 when I started getting hair on my face and down below and then had my first wet dream. I was worried that there was something wrong with me because no one ever said anything about that sort of stuff.

Brian, 18

I started getting hair on my balls and round my cock. It wasn't much of a surprise because we'd had sex education lessons at school which I suppose were kind of useful.

Darwen, 19

I was a late developer and nothing happened until I was about 15 or 16. I was worried by that time, but my mum had tried to reassure me, even though other kids at school kept winding me up because I was different.

Aaron, 21

*One guy at school grew much faster than everyone
else and got hair on his face and things. He got teased,
but that's probably because he was a bit of an arsehole
anyway. Mind you, we were careful how much we
teased him because he was a lot bigger than us!*

Mark, 18

When Does It Happen?

Everyone goes through puberty – but it can start at different times in different people. And what happens to you probably won't be exactly the same as what happens to your friends. The first sign of puberty is usually when your testes and then your penis start to get larger. In most boys this happens between the ages of 10 and 14 – the most common age is 12. A few months later you'll start to notice pubic hair growing around your penis. About two years after you've noticed the first changes you'll have your main growth spurt – this is when you're growing fastest. The most common age for this is just under 14.

It often seems that boys start puberty much later than girls, but this is not actually true. In girls, the changes (such as breast development) are more obvious to the outside world and they tend to do most of their growing early on in puberty, while boys have their main growth spurt later. This is why many 11- and 12-year-old girls are taller than boys of the same age. By 16 most of the girls have stopped growing and the boys have overtaken them.

What Changes Should I Expect?

This is a picture of a boy who is about halfway through the changes of puberty:

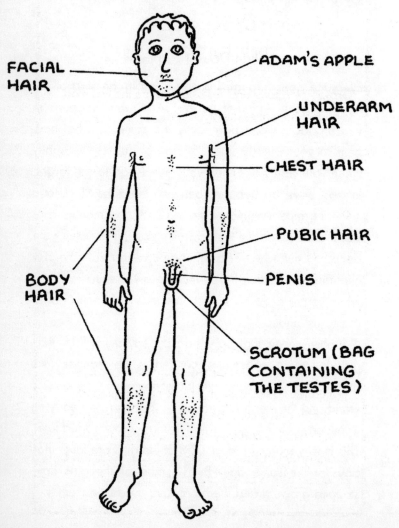

FACIAL HAIR

ADAM'S APPLE

UNDERARM HAIR

CHEST HAIR

PUBIC HAIR

PENIS

BODY HAIR

SCROTUM (BAG CONTAINING THE TESTES)

Perhaps you are taller or shorter, fatter or thinner or have more or less body hair than this boy. However, the changes in this picture will apply to you at some stage too.

DOC BOX
Important Hormones

Growth Hormone and *Testosterone* are the two most important hormones during puberty.

Growth Hormone is:
◇ produced by the pituitary gland at the base of the brain
◇ vital for growth
◇ at its highest levels in children and young adults
◇ usually produced nightly by your body shortly after you've fallen into deep sleep

Testosterone is:
◇ the male sex hormone
◇ produced by your testes
◇ responsible for increase in body hair, voice change, development of sexual organs and sperm and sexual behaviour. (NB: These are all called secondary male characteristics.)
◇ important in speeding up muscle development and the rate at which your body works

What Causes Puberty?

Puberty and the changes that take place in your body are controlled by *hormones*. A hormone is like a chemical messenger. It is made in one part of the body (usually a gland) and then, using the bloodstream as a transport system, it travels all over your body delivering instructions, which control how your body works and develops. Hormone production doesn't just happen during puberty. You were producing hormones before you were born and you'll go on producing them throughout your life.

Changes in Body Size and Shape

You often notice your growth spurt first in your feet, when your shoes suddenly feel too small. Your feet are the first things to start growing, quickly followed by your arms, legs and hands. At the peak of your growth spurt your height could be increasing by over 11 cm a year and this can make you feel awkward and clumsy. Suddenly your arms and legs are longer and it's easy to knock into or trip over things.

I kept tripping up stairs. At the time I couldn't work out why, but there was this one particular staircase at school and I was always falling when I ran up it. It was like my legs and feet didn't do what they were supposed to do any more.

Peter, 19

I remember when I started growing people and things seemed to knock into me a lot. My mum got really cross because I turned round and knocked over her favourite ornament with my elbow. Later, when she'd calmed down, she said she realised I couldn't help it and it was probably just because I was growing so fast.

Stephen, 17

Most boys grow upwards before they grow outwards. Your shoulders won't begin to broaden until you're about halfway through puberty. Around the same time your muscles will begin to develop, particularly in your arms, legs and chest. This makes you stronger and you may notice a real difference, particularly if you play sport. Some boys want to push this and start training hard to increase their muscle growth. This is not necessary and could even be dangerous.

As you grow taller your weight will increase as well. But when your muscles begin to develop you'll notice that you become even heavier. This is because muscle weighs more than bone or fat. Many boys find their body shape changes quite dramatically during puberty and some of them worry that they might be becoming too thin or too fat. The best person to advise you on this is your school nurse or family doctor and there's more information about diet and weight in Chapter 5.

Another problem that worries many boys is an increase in the size of their breasts. Part of this is due to the development of muscles and fat around the chest,

25

DOC BOX
Dangers of Over-Training

Training too often (more than four times a week) or too hard (for long periods of time or at a very high intensity level) can cause problems in some boys. Your bones and ligaments are still growing and damage can occur at the join between the two. This is called *osteochondritis*. In can happen in several areas, such as in the knees, feet and back, and it's very painful. If it happens in your knee, the only treatment is to rest the leg – usually in a plaster cast – for several weeks.

The other main danger associated with training too hard is dehydration. If you exercise for more than half an hour (or less than that, if it's hot) you must remember to drink – little and often. Water, dilute squash or special sports drinks are all ideal. You can check whether you're drinking enough by looking at the colour of your urine (pee) after you finish exercising. It should be a pale, straw colour – if it's dark yellow or orange, you haven't drunk enough. Top athletes know their performance really suffers if they are dehydrated – and yours will too!

but changing hormones can sometimes cause breast development on one or both sides. If this happens to you, don't worry – it's perfectly normal and usually goes away. In the very rare cases when breasts don't go back to normal it's possible to have surgery to deal with the problem.

DOC BOX
Steroids and 'Growth Inducers'

Anabolic steroids are powerful drugs similar to the male sex hormone, testosterone. They are dangerous and rarely prescribed by doctors, but they are sometimes used illegally in sports and body-building to develop muscle and strength.

Steroids and growth inducers have serious side effects, including:

◇ acne
◇ shrinking of testes
◇ problems with erection
◇ inability to produce sperm
◇ liver cancer
◇ heart attacks
◇ strokes

continued on next page

They can also cause aggression and depression. They can increase muscle strength, but the tendons and ligaments which anchor the muscles to the joints don't become stronger, so you may get long-term injuries. If you start using them as a teenager, they may stop you growing to your full height.

Creatine is a chemical substance which is used mainly by body-builders to add muscle bulk. It is usually sold as a dietary supplement. Manufacturers claim that it allows you to exercise at a harder level for longer. It does result in more water being stored in muscle cells so muscles can appear bigger; however, there is not really any good scientific evidence that it has much effect on actual muscle power. It can cause damage to the kidneys if you take too much.

If you want to build muscles safely, you should get some advice from a good gym or sports coach, rather than taking any supplements.

Body Hair

One of the early signs of puberty is the growth of hair under your arms and above your penis. At first there may only be one or two straggly hairs, but these quickly increase and you'll also find more hair on your legs and the backs of your hands. Facial hair doesn't usually start showing until after your body hair has increased. At first it's often light and wispy and it may take months before you need to shave every day. For more information on shaving see Chapter 5.

Some boys also grow chest hair during puberty, but it may not develop until years later and even then, not all men have it.

Spots and Smells

There are also some less welcome signs of puberty. The oil glands in your skin become more active, often leading to spots and acne. Taking care to keep your face clean and using special oil-control washes and products can help, but you can also ask the pharmacist or your GP for advice (see Chapter 5).

Sweat glands also become more active – not just those under your arms, but also those on the soles of your feet, the palms of your hands and even between your legs. You produce more sweat and it smells stronger. And if you let it get stale it becomes very unpleasant indeed. You need a bath or shower plus clean underwear every day.

Voice Breaking

During puberty the male hormone, testosterone, makes your voice box (larynx) at the front of the neck grow larger and change shape. You'll notice this in two ways. Your Adam's apple – the round bit at the front of your neck that bobs up and down when you swallow –

becomes more obvious and your voice gets deeper. This can happen very suddenly – almost overnight – or take place gradually over a few weeks or months. It can feel as if your voice is all over the place – high and squeaky one minute and low and gruff the next. Unfortunately there's very little you can do to control this and it always seems to squeak at the wrong moment. It's also very obvious to everyone around you and a common cause for teasing. This may be upsetting, but remember that it's a sign you're growing up and some boys may just be jealous it's happening to you before it happens to them.

The worst bit about puberty is when you have the piss taken out of you because your voice is breaking. There's nothing quite as embarrassing as when it suddenly goes very high – usually at the worst possible moment, like when you're trying to chat someone up. One guy I knew had it happen during a school play. It took ages for him to live it down.   Ed, 18

My voice broke in literally one week when I was on holiday. My brothers took the piss like mad when I got home and my parents were really embarrassing when they tried to say something tactful and supportive about it. But I know everyone feels like this. You just have to get over it.   Mark, 18

I didn't really notice anything until I was about 13 or 14. Then my voice broke. I just woke up one morning and it had gone deep, right down to my boots. Everyone takes the mick but it's a rite of passage and something you want to go through.   Geoff, 25

Delayed Puberty

Although there's a big variation in the age when puberty happens, about 1 in 100 teenage boys have delayed puberty. This usually means no signs at all of puberty – no change in growth, body hair or genital size – by the age of 14. It often runs in families, and it doesn't need any kind of treatment, as development takes place normally in the next year or so. But sometimes severe illness, hormone problems or being very underweight can cause delayed puberty.

If you and/or your parents are worried you should talk to your family doctor. He/she may refer you to a paediatrician (a specialist young people's doctor). The paediatrician will ask questions about your general health and what age the rest of your family started puberty. They might do an X-ray and blood tests and can usually reassure you that everything is normal. In the rare case where there is a real problem they might offer a short course (usually a few months) of hormone treatment to get puberty started. This should be enough to kick-start your own natural hormones so that they take over and complete the process.

I was really worried because I was the only boy in Year 10 who hadn't got any hair under my arms or on my face. I was 14½ and felt really stupid. Although I had been one of the tall ones in junior school, everyone was overtaking me – I was even smaller than some of the girls. Some of them were quite nice – one girl kept saying I was 'small and sweet' – but I felt so embarrassed. One day I blurted it all out to my mum and she offered to come to see my GP with me for a check-up. He talked to us together for a few minutes and asked me some questions about how healthy I was and if I was taking any medicines. He was interested in the fact that my dad had told me that he had been a 'late developer' too. Then he gave me a check-up on my own. He showed me my height and weight on a chart and then compared the size of my testicles with some funny wooden beads to check whether they'd started to grow yet. He was able to tell me that they had begun to develop and he also noticed that I was starting to get some very fine hairs at the base of my penis. He said that things were about to start happening and I shouldn't worry. He also explained that just before the start of puberty you actually grow very slowly.

I went back six months later for a check-up and by then I knew that everything was OK. I had started to grow in height at last, and my testes were bigger as well as my penis. A great relief!

My doctor said that if he hadn't seen any signs of puberty when he examined me the first time he would have sent me to see a hospital specialist, as most boys do have some changes by around 14. At the hospital they *might have done some blood tests and, depending on what they showed, they could have given me a drug to start puberty off.*   John, 16

Problem Page

I'm 13 and really worried because I think I'm growing breasts. I felt them in the shower and one's bigger than the other – it feels like a big grape. It's really sore too. I won't be able to have showers at school any more as my mates will think I'm turning into a girl!

Don't panic! This is called *gynaecomastia* – a fancy word meaning breast development in boys. Almost every boy gets it at some stage as he goes through puberty. It's caused by a hormone called *oestrogen* which occurs in the blood in both boys and girls. The male sex hormone levels eventually get higher than the oestrogen levels in boys and stop any further growth of the breasts. It is very rare for the problem to carry on but it can last for up to two years.

Is there any easy way to calculate how tall I will be?

Tallness (or shortness) usually runs in families and you can use your parents' height to give you a rough idea of how tall you'll be when you're fully grown. Your final height will be the average of your parents' measurements (add your mum and dad's heights together and divide by two) plus or minus 9 cm.

Your school nurse or doctor can give you a more accurate prediction by plotting your parents' heights on a special chart and comparing the size you are now against it.

I'm sure there's something wrong with me because everyone else seems to have started puberty. I'm 13 and nothing's happened and I'm sick of my friends boasting about how big their privates are because I know they're really laughing at me.

Most boys will have noticed some signs, such as hairs under their arms or round their penis by the time they're 14, but a few won't start puberty until a year or two later. However, if you do start late, there's a chance that the process will happen quite suddenly, so you'll catch up with and maybe even overtake some of your friends. In the meantime try to ignore their boasting and teasing. It might help to remember that boys often make fun of someone when they're feeling insecure about their own bodies. Perhaps some of the boasting you're hearing is more wishful thinking than truth!

My voice has been breaking for a few weeks now but sometimes it still goes really squeaky, especially if I'm nervous. What can I do to control it?

It can take months for your voice to settle down, but even grown men can sound a bit high pitched and squeaky when they're feeling worried or anxious. Anxiety makes your breathing faster and more shallow and your muscles tense, including the ones surrounding your voice box. This is what causes the squeakiness. Learning to relax and breathing deeply and slowly can help open up your voice box, making your voice sound deeper and more resonant. If you have to give a talk or presentation you can use an actors' trick of chewing gum or yawning a lot just before you have to speak. This can also help to relax your voice and upper body making your speech clearer.

I dread games lessons at school because I hate getting changed in public. Most of the other boys don't seem to mind at all and parade around without anything on. But I'm sure they're all looking at me and secretly laughing.

Maybe some of the boys really aren't as confident as they look. Others will be secretly worrying that people are looking at them too. At your age there's a huge variation in stages of development and it's easy to feel self-conscious in public if you started puberty later than your friends. But it doesn't mean there's anything wrong with you. And it's your own nervousness that's making you more aware of the differences. Anyone else who points them out or tries to make fun of you is almost certainly trying to cover up their own insecurities or the fear that you – and everyone else – is secretly laughing at *them*!

Chapter 3

Puberty: Willies & Private Parts

This chapter covers:
- ◇ Development of private parts
- ◇ Size and shape of penis
- ◇ Circumcision
- ◇ Mechanics of erection
- ◇ Mechanics of sperm production
- ◇ Orgasm and ejaculation
- ◇ Wet dreams and erections
- ◇ Masturbation

When we were researching this book we asked boys what question they would most like to put (in private) to a doctor who specialised in young people's problems. You may not be very surprised to learn that two questions appeared more than any other:

- ◇ At what age should my private parts start growing?
- ◇ How big should my penis be?

In this chapter we answer these questions and many more by talking about the average age when changes happen. Averages are always worked out by looking at hundreds of people – but you have to remember that lots of them will fall on one side or the other of the average figure. So don't worry if you don't notice all the changes at exactly the ages mentioned here – you're still perfectly normal!

When Will My Private Parts Start to Get Bigger?

The first thing you might notice is your testes getting bigger. The skin of the scrotum starts to look darker – and a bit reddish – and gets rougher and thicker. At around the same time your penis begins to grow. First it gets a bit longer, then, after about a year, it becomes a bit broader.

You're most likely to notice your genitals (private parts) growing around the age of 11 to 12, but some boys develop very early (as young as 8 or 9), while others may be later (16 or 17).

About six months after your testes start to get bigger, pubic hair begins to grow. At first it is fair and quite straight, usually around the base of the penis. Over the next few months it will get darker, coarser and more curly and spread over the whole pubic area. Eventually it grows upwards in the middle towards your tummy button or *umbilicus* and may stretch round behind your testes towards your bottom or anus.

The average boy will have finished developing by around 15, but if you're one of the ones who doesn't start puberty until later, your genitals might carry on growing until you're 18 or 19.

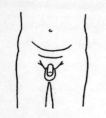

PENIS AND TESTICLES
OF A CHILD

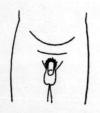

FIRST SIGNS OF PUBERTY—
PUBIC HAIR STARTS TO APPEAR,
TESTES GET LARGER BUT PENIS
IS STILL THE SAME SIZE

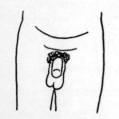

PENIS GROWS LONGER
AND WIDER. GLANS
(HEAD) MORE DEVELOPED.
TESTICLES GET LARGER
AND PUBIC HAIR INCREASES.

When I was 10 or 11, I thought my penis would never grow and that I'd never be able to have sex because it would always be too small. My friends made it worse by telling me that wearing Y-fronts prevent you from developing properly down below. They all reckoned they had 6 inch willies and balls like balloons! There was a lot of mickey taking of the late-starters (like me) who had no pubic hair. Luckily everything began doing what it was supposed to do when I was about 12.

Mark, 15

The worst thing for me about growing up was that there were other boys who were clearly more developed much sooner. Communal sports changing rooms were a nightmare. I felt everyone was looking at me and wondered if I'd be some kind of a freak, stuck with a kid's body forever. I didn't really hit puberty until I was 14 but then everything happened at once.

Baz, 21

38

I started growing quite a thick, hairy chest at about 14. Although I'm proud of it now it was quite embarrassing in the showers after a PE lesson. Most of my mates hadn't even started puberty and there was me looking like their dads!

Toby, 19

How Big Should My Penis Be?

This is probably a source of concern for boys and men all over the world! It's made much worse by some people's exaggerated boasting as well as porn films which tend to feature men who are definitely larger than normal – possibly due to cosmetic surgery or clever camera angles!

Most fully grown penises measure between 12 and 18 cm (about 5–7 inches) in length when fully erect. Of course you can usually increase this measurement a bit if you dig the ruler or tape measure deeper into your flesh at the base of your penis! The most common length is between 15 and 16½ cm (6–6½ inches). The average circumference – presumably measured around the fattest part of the erect penis – is between 11½ and 14 cm (4½–5½ inches).

TRY NOT TO WORRY

But penises are very unpredictable. One that looks quite big while it's limp or flaccid might not actually grow much larger on erection. Others can look quite small but grow much more on erection.

Everyone worries about their length but you've got to learn that there can be too much of a good thing – it really is quality over quantity! I found reading the sex columns in women's magazines invaluable. You learn that boys always exaggerate and most of their myths are about 'measuring up'.   Daniel, 16

My parents never said much, but my older brother bought me a book about growing up. It was helpful but I was still worried that I wouldn't be big enough to satisfy women. That's still a fear for me, because I'm sure it's just below average. But my girlfriend has made me more confident. I haven't slept with her but she says it's 'big'. I think she's just trying to stop me from worrying.   James, 16

I was expecting my penis to grow but I couldn't quite imagine what it would be like. One day I was in my room sort of playing with myself (not even masturbating because I didn't really know what it was I was doing) and I had my first orgasm and discharge. This completely stunned me. Almost immediately my penis started getting bigger and for a while I thought I'd damaged it by playing with myself.   J, 17

What Shape Should It Be?

Some penises are long and thin, others are short and fat. And although they all point upwards when they get hard and excited (if yours doesn't you should check it out with your doctor), some of them also curve a little bit to the

40

right or left or up or down. As long as your penis doesn't hurt when it gets hard and erect there's no need to worry if it isn't 100% straight.

Circumcised and Uncircumcised

Another thing that affects how a penis looks is whether or not it's circumcised.

An uncircumcised or natural penis has a sleeve of skin called the *foreskin*, which protects its head or *glans* and gives it a pointed appearance in its normal, non-erect state.

Circumcision is an operation to remove the foreskin, so a circumcised penis has a rounded rather than pointed end because the head is always exposed.

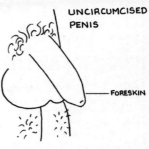

Although a circumcised and uncircumcised penis may look very different when they're just hanging in their floppy state, when they become erect it's hard to tell them apart. This is because when an uncircumcised penis becomes erect, the foreskin is pushed back (sometimes with a little help) over the head leaving it rounded and exposed.

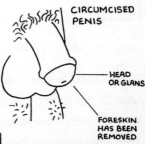

Circumcision is usually carried

41

out on babies or very young boys as a religious or cultural custom, but sometimes young boys and (very rarely) young men have it done for health reasons. Many religious groups, including Jews and Muslims as well as some African tribes, circumcise baby boys. In America the majority of men are circumcised, but it is a lot less common in the UK. People used to think that a circumcised penis was cleaner than an uncircumcised one, but this is not the case. It is true that *smegma* can collect under the foreskin and get very smelly, but as long as you remember to pull back your foreskin and clean yourself carefully and regularly, this should not be a problem.

DOC BOX
What Is Smegma?

Smegma is soft, white, cheesy stuff produced by tiny glands on the inside of the foreskin. It collects in the creases under the foreskin and, if you don't keep yourself clean, can occasionally become infected making it smelly and sticky.

Medical Reasons for Circumcision

Some teenage boys and men find their foreskins are too tight. This condition is called *para-phimosis*. It means the foreskin cannot be pulled back over the glans of the penis. This makes sex or masturbation very sore, so a doctor might recommend circumcision. It will be carried out under a general anaesthetic (so you're fast asleep and can't feel anything). The operation removes the whole foreskin, but takes only a few minutes and is usually done as a 'day-case' so you don't have to stay overnight in hospital.

All the men in our family are circumcised and my older brother told me these horror tales about showers at school where people will point you out and laugh. I dreaded going up to senior school for that reason but, although I felt self-conscious that I was different, no one ever said anything – not to my face anyway.   David, 17

I was circumcised when I was very small and when I was growing up it really worried me that my penis wouldn't be big enough because of it. For a while I was also scared I would damage myself by masturbating because there was no foreskin to protect it. Now I know that neither of these things are true – and it all seems to have turned out OK.   Tom, 18

The Mechanics of Erection

Your penis is made of spongy tissue with a small tube, the *urethra*, running through it. Urine (pee) and semen (the liquid containing sperm) both come out through the urethra – but not at the same time.

When you become sexually excited, extra blood flows into your penis filling up the spongy tissue. At the same time muscles tighten around the base of the penis to stop

43

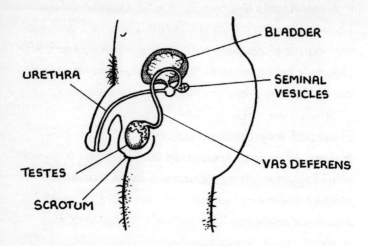

BLADDER

URETHRA

SEMINAL
VESICLES

VAS DEFERENS

TESTES

SCROTUM

too much blood flowing out again so the penis gets stiff and begins to stand out from your body. Because of all the extra blood, it will also feel warmer and may look darker in colour, particularly at the end around the glans.

The Mechanics of Sperm Production

Most boys have two testes (although you can manage perfectly well with one). Testes produce *sperm* and male sex hormones, and they lie in a sac of skin called the *scrotum* which hangs down between your legs. Having your testes outside the main part of your body keeps them cooler, which is good for sperm production. In fact men who wear tight trousers or pants tend to make fewer sperm than those who wear loose boxers!

It takes 70 to 80 days for a sperm to develop fully. Each mature sperm has a fat head and a long tail – a bit like a tadpole.

A sperm looks like this:

HEAD

. . . except of course it's much smaller. Their tails help them to swim once they are inside your sexual partner's body.

When the sperm are fully developed they travel up through the *vas deferens* or sperm duct to a holding area just below your bladder where they wait until they are ejaculated.

FLAGELLUM (TAIL)

A SPERM

Semen

Semen is the liquid that comes out of your penis when you reach an orgasm and ejaculate. It contains sperm plus some extra liquid produced by different glands in the male sex organs. The largest part of it comes from the *seminal vesicles* – small sex glands near the end of the vas deferens just before it joins the urethra or urine tube (see diagram). This part of the semen contains lots of sugar, giving the sperm an energy boost

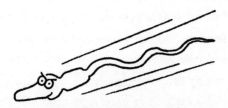

IT'S SUPERSPERM! FASTER THAN A SPEEDING BULLET!

45

which starts them thrashing their tails and moving more quickly, ready to make their journey in search of a female egg.

Orgasm and Ejaculation

Ejaculation is when the semen shoots out of the end of the penis. It is the orgasm or climax – the high point of sexual arousal. Several things happen during orgasm and ejaculation:

◇ First the semen is produced and mixes with the sperm.

◇ At around the same time, a valve at the top of the urethra closes to stop urine coming out from the bladder.

◇ The muscle fibres in the scrotum contract, pulling the testes up towards your body.

◇ Your heartbeat and breathing get faster.

◇ Your blood pressure increases.

◇ The skin on your face or chest may get flushed or reddish.

◇ Your nipples may become hard, stand out more and feel extremely sensitive.

◇ The glans or head of your penis may darken to a red or purple colour.

◇ One or two drops of clear or milky fluid may appear at the end of your penis.

◇ Finally (and all of this can happen very quickly) the muscles in and around your penis start to contract, pushing the semen out of your body, along your urethra until it spurts out at the end of your penis – usually in 3 or 4 bursts. This is often called *coming*.

An orgasm is a bit like sneezing – although it feels much, much better than that! Just beforehand there's a point where you know that, whatever you do, it is going to happen. Your body tenses up, then goes into a final spasm of sensation which centres on your penis. Afterwards you feel very relaxed or sleepy. Your heartbeat and breathing gradually go back to normal and your penis goes soft again as you lose your erection.

Your body usually needs a resting time before you can have another erection, but this can be anything from a few minutes to several hours – or even a day or more. Older men often find it takes a lot longer for them to recover!

The Penis With a Mind of Its Own

Although babies and young boys often get erections – and obviously enjoy touching and playing with themselves – you might not have your first ejaculation until you're 13 or 14. Often this is in the form of a *wet dream*. During the night it's normal for your penis to grow hard and then soft again several times over. And it's very common to wake up with an erection. Sometimes things go further and during the night you ejaculate – without even knowing about it. In the morning you find a wet or sticky patch on your pyjamas or the bedclothes. You might even wonder if you've wet the bed. We don't know whether this sort of sleeping ejaculation is always linked to sexy dreams or not. Most people don't remember many of their dreams anyway. What we do know is that wet dreams are beyond your control. There's nothing you can do to stop them.

Wet dreams were a real problem – especially in my middle teens. No one ever explained about them and I never asked questions. I hid the evidence and kind of worked it out for myself what was going on. I enjoyed waking up with erections, though – almost looked forward to it.
                                                                Jim, 25

Amazing Body Facts

◇ A sperm is only 0.05 mm long – 200 sperm laid end to end would only be 1 cm long

◇ A sperm can swim about 3 mm an hour, or about 7 cm in 24 hours

◇ Approximately 500,000,000 sperm are made every day by a healthy adult man

◇ The amount of semen produced is related to age, plus how long it has been since you last ejaculated. Average volume is between 2 and 7 mls (½ –1½ tsp.)

My big problem was wet dreams. It was too difficult to ask someone what was happening, but it was like waking up in a waterbed. I lived with my dad, so I just washed my own stuff, but I can't imagine what it would have been like if I'd had to tell my mum what was going on.

Geoff, 25

I remember being very worried about how I'd explain it to my mum. Luckily when it did happen she didn't say anything at all, probably because I had an older brother so she'd seen it all before. Josh, 19

But of course erections don't only happen during the night. During puberty your penis can seem to develop a

◇ Each ml of semen contains a huge number of sperm – around 10 to 20,000,000 – and it only takes one to fertilise an egg!

◇ The sperm can carry on swimming for a long time after they are ejaculated – half will still be moving after two hours and some can keep going a lot longer

◇ Semen can be thin and runny or sticky and thick, yellow or white. What you eat can affect how it looks or smells

mind of its own, reacting instantly to the slightest hint of sex. It could be something on TV, seeing a girl you like at school, a dirty joke or a newspaper ad. Sometimes there's no obvious reason at all. You're sitting there minding your own business and whoops, suddenly there's an erection. This can be embarrassing and can make you a target for teasing, but you should know that it's normal and healthy – and happens to everyone.

I often seemed to get hard-ons in class, especially if I was bored. It was as though my mind wandered and the blood all drained away from my brain. They were a nightmare, especially if there was a possibility of being asked to stand up and read a passage from a book or something. Girls have no idea what we have to cope with!
Baz, 21

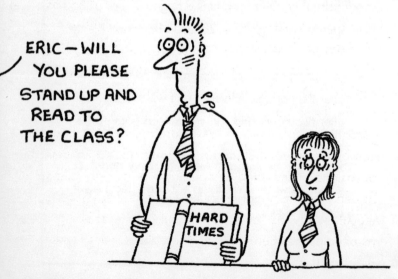

ERIC – WILL YOU PLEASE STAND UP AND READ TO THE CLASS?

HARD TIMES

I was always very careful to take my school bag everywhere with me just in case I got a hard-on during the day as I needed to hold it in front of my body at those vital moments. I suppose I was quite resourceful, really!

James, 20

Probably the worst times for me were in the showers at school. I was terrified of getting an erection in front of the other boys. I knew they'd think I was gay (I wasn't) but it was almost as if the fear of it happening made it even more likely.

Simon, 18.

Masturbation

Masturbation means touching or playing with your sexual parts to give yourself pleasure. People used to think it was evil or dangerous or would cause all kinds of conditions, like blindness or insanity. Some religions and cultures still have a taboo against it. However, most doctors and experts now agree that not only is it safe, it's also a positively healthy, normal way to explore your own body and its sexual arousal. Of course it's still a subject for many dirty jokes and it's something you should only ever do in private, but you can be fairly sure that most boys do it. For some it's an occasional comforting thing they do before falling asleep. They may not even masturbate all the way to ejaculation. Other boys go through phases of doing it as often as they can – and thinking about it even when they can't!

Many boys like to fantasise about things when they masturbate. It might be about a girl they like, a singer or actress they have a crush on or some kind of complicated sexual fantasy that they would never admit to anyone else. Many feel guilty about doing this, but it's important to realise that fantasy is very different from reality.

Some boys masturbate with other boys. They may enjoy watching each other doing it, compete to see who can get there fastest or ejaculate the farthest, or even touch each other's penises to see what it feels like. Adults are often shocked by this and boys can worry it means they are homosexual or gay. But this sort of sex play is fairly common when boys are growing up and doesn't usually have any connection with whether they are gay or straight.

Problem Page

I'm worried about my balls. Sometimes they hang much higher than other times. I notice it particularly when I'm getting changed after games at school. I hate other people seeing my body and it makes me feel as though my balls are shrivelling up.

Your balls or testes hang in a sac of skin, called the scrotum, between your legs. This has a clever built-in device for protecting the developing sperm which need to be kept at a temperature a few degrees lower than your body. Most of the time the scrotum hangs loose allowing the testes to stay cool. But sometimes, particularly if you're cold, the muscles in the wall of the scrotum tighten and thicken, drawing the testes up closer towards the body, keeping them warmer. The same thing happens if you're scared or nervous – which probably explains why you feel like this getting changed in public. It might help to remember that other boys are just as self-conscious and, if they tease you or make unkind comments, it's often just an attempt to divert attention from themselves.

I sometimes get a hard-on at the worst possible moment – usually when I'm talking to a girl. Or even when I'm watching TV with my parents. Once it happened in a swimming lesson at school and I was scared to get out of the pool in case everyone noticed. What can I do about this?

All boys suffer from this and, to some extent, it's a matter of learning to live with it. Hard-ons (erections) will go away after a while, although they may leave your penis and testes feeling achy for a bit. This is a result of the increased blood flow to your penis and the surrounding areas during sexual arousal and erection. Thinking about something completely non-sexual or even frightening will sometimes help the erection wilt more quickly. Some boys resort to wearing tighter underpants (or even two pairs) to stop it being obvious. However, this isn't very good for you as it can increase the temperature of the testes and decrease sperm production. When it happens in the swimming pool your best bet is to 'suddenly decide' that you're going to swim another few lengths. You won't be the first boy to use this excuse!

I often masturbate several times a day and I'm worried that I will run out of sperm. Is this likely?

Your body makes about 500,000,000 sperm every day so there's no way you're going to run out. However, if you do masturbate several times in a day there will be fewer sperm in the later ejaculations. But a few hours' rest or sleep will build up the store again.

I'm really worried about masturbating. Although I do it, I'm scared because I've heard that it can be addictive and ruin your chances of enjoying sex later on.

Many boys and young men masturbate a great deal. It's normal and healthy as long as it doesn't interfere with the rest of their lives. And many men continue to masturbate occasionally or frequently, even when they have a regular sexual partner. There is a slight risk that you can become used to the very rough handling you might be giving your penis so, when you start to have sex, the sensation of intercourse might not feel sufficiently stimulating. But the excitement of making love with another person usually over-comes this problem and most men realise that making love and masturbation are two completely different things.

Is pornography bad for you? I know most grown-ups wouldn't approve, but I do find it exciting to look at magazines and pictures on the internet.

One of the sexual differences between men and women is that men are more easily aroused by pictures of nudity (nakedness) or people having sex. It's common for boys and men to use these pictures or videos as a stimulus for masturbation. But you need to be aware that many people do find this offensive and upsetting. Girlfriends and wives often see it as men being unfaithful, although their men don't view it as anything that might harm their relationships. The real problem comes when you start relying on harder or more violent pornography to become aroused. Because of the internet this is more widely available than ever before and there is a danger that you could begin to see sexual partners as objects to be used or hurt, rather than as equals in a loving relationship. Pornography can certainly become addictive because it gives such an easy thrill. Real life means dealing with real people and their emotions. This can seem like hard work compared to your magazines or websites. If this sounds familiar then it's certainly time to cut back on the porn and concentrate on girls as people and potential friends.

Chapter 4

Emotional Pressures & Changes

This chapter covers:
- ◇ How hormones can affect your emotions
- ◇ Dealing with anger and aggression
- ◇ Problems with parents
- ◇ Sex on the brain
- ◇ Am I gay?
- ◇ Self-confidence
- ◇ Depression and suicide

Puberty doesn't just make you look different – you feel different too. The same hormones which are speeding up your growth and development are affecting your emotions. Some of this is hard to miss. Because one of the major hormones is testosterone, the male sex hormone, your brain starts to become very interested in sex – in fact you might feel you can't think about anything else! But some of the other emotional changes are less obvious.

When I was about 13, I started having these colossal mood swings. My parents weren't sympathetic. They compared me to Harry Enfield's Kevin. Totally unfair! The only way out of it was to shut myself away in my room for a while because it would seem like the whole world was against me. Then I'd put it back in perspective and wonder what all the fuss was about.   Tom, 20

My relationship with my parents changed when I was 10. They seemed to think I was moody when personally I didn't think I'd done anything wrong. This really got to me. Mum kept on saying things like, 'You've got an attitude problem' when I'd hardly said anything. It gives you a very hollow feeling and makes you feel patronised. It seems like everyone is against you, even though you've done nothing wrong. My way of coping was to go into my room and listen to music. That's how I got into rap music. It's kinda 'retaliation' music.   James, 16

When I got to 12 or 13, I always seemed to feel annoyed. It didn't matter what people did, I still felt cross.
          Cleeton, 16

I was very moody from 13 to 15, but I grew out of it. I'd pick on my sister or shout for no reason. I was evil towards my mum at some points, but my dad sorted me out! Looking back I can't explain why I was so moody and nasty. I just couldn't help it.   Mark, 18

I became more independent and much more distant. I stopped confiding in my mum regarding worries about personal stuff. I had strong opinions and I wouldn't listen to anyone else's view.   Richard, 17

DOC BOX
The Effects of Testosterone

The male sex hormone, testosterone, is produced by the testes, but has effects all over the body – including the brain! The amount produced increases from about the age of 8, peaks at between 20 and 30, and then falls slowly. It is the main hormone responsible for the male sex drive and 'normal' male aggression. It also causes:

◇ growth and development of all the bones in the skeleton
◇ development of muscle

Aggression

As you go through puberty you grow bigger, and more muscular and powerful, but you can also lose your temper more easily. You might feel the urge to lash out when there's nothing obviously wrong. Being stuck halfway between childhood and adulthood is frustrating and you want things to happen faster. You want them to happen NOW. You might feel that other people, such as parents or teachers, don't take you seriously, or expect too much from you one moment and then treat you like a child the next. When frustration builds up it can explode into anger.

◇ growth of beard as well as pubic, underarm
  and body hair
◇ deepening of the voice
◇ increase in size of the penis, testes and scrotum
◇ later in life, gradual baldness with loss of hair at
  front and sides of head

Although testosterone is an important part of being a male, too much is definitely a bad thing! Athletes, who sometimes take testosterone illegally to try to improve their performance, can end up with:

◇ severe aggressive behaviour
◇ mood swings
◇ liver tumours (cancer)

Aggression and violence have always played a part in male culture and we know that men often prefer to act rather than talk, whereas women often prefer to talk. Some of this is due to chemical differences in the brain. But it's not as simple as that. Although men and women are obviously biologically different, our society also pro-grammes them to be different. Adults react differently towards baby boys and baby girls. They tend to play rough and tumble, loud and more aggressive games with boys, but act more gently and quietly with girls.

The way you behave and the way you expect people

to behave towards you isn't just controlled by your hormones and your biology, but by the way your parents and everyone else have treated you throughout your life.

Dealing With Anger

Everyone gets angry sometimes – it's part of being human. And, the less control you feel you have over your life, the more frustrated and angry you are likely to become. During adolescence, the growing-up period, it can feel as though everyone's getting at you but no one is listening. Pressures build up at home and school; your teachers are on your back because you're late with coursework, your mum is nagging you about the state of your room and your best mate suddenly gets a girlfriend and doesn't have time for you. You're upset, you're angry and you want to lash out. Anger is destructive. But that doesn't mean you shouldn't feel it. The question is what to do about it!

There are two important things to learn about anger:

◇ Finding a way of getting rid of some of the immediate angry feelings makes it less likely you'll explode.
◇ Learning to talk about the things that are making you angry can help people to understand.

If you can master these two points you'll be a lot happier, infinitely more popular with everyone and you stand a much better chance of getting what YOU want.

Reducing Angry Feelings

There are many ways of coping with even the worst feelings of anger. Not all of them work all of the time, so experiment to find the best strategy for you.

⬦ Sport – whether playing in a football match or just going for a run or a swim. This releases chemicals into the bloodstream that give you a natural high, reducing the sensation of frustration and aggression.

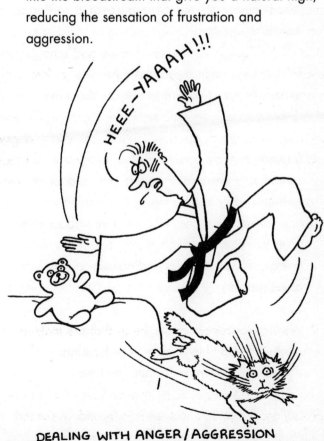

DEALING WITH ANGER / AGGRESSION

◇ Thumping a pillow or a cushion. This is a 'safe' way of being aggressive and, although it might sound silly, it does make you feel a lot better.

◇ Playing music. Losing yourself in your favourite type of sound helps you gain some distance, calm down and bring your emotions back into line. But if part of the problem is your mum nagging you about loud music, it's probably best to wear headphones!

◇ Talking to someone who understands – your mum or best friend or a helpline like ChildLine (see Chapter 9 for more helplines).

◇ Learning to walk away. This is a tricky one, but it's remarkably effective. If people are used to you getting mad or lashing out, simply turning your back and walking away will take them by surprise. It also gives you time to see things in perspective before going back more calmly and explaining your side of the problem.

◇ Writing down your feelings – in a diary, story or poem. You don't ever have to show it to anyone but putting it down on paper can help.

◇ Crying. It may not be seen as very manly, but recent research suggests that crying is an excellent way of coping with strong emotion. It seems that crying when you are genuinely upset helps reduce some of the chemicals which cause the brain to experience anxiety, anger and depression. So you genuinely do feel better afterwards.

Talking About the Things That Make You Angry

Once you've coped with your immediate feelings you should be able to go back and express whatever it was that made you so angry in a clear and calm way. This gets your message across effectively and gives you a better chance of achieving whatever it is you want.

◇ If you did lose your temper, start off by apologising. It doesn't cost you anything and it disarms the other person, whether it's your mum, teacher, girlfriend or best mate.

◇ Work out before you start exactly what it is that's making you so upset and what needs to change in order for you to feel better.

◇ Put it as simply and directly as possible, – I feel really angry/hurt/upset/unloved when you . . . (then be prepared to give specific examples).

◇ Next (and very important) listen to what the other person has to say.

◇ Then make a suggestion. Maybe it's a matter of your mum understanding that you can't clean your room until the end of the week because you're so behind with your coursework. Or that next time your friend has to cancel an arrangement, it would be better if they rang to tell you rather than just not turn up. Make a positive, constructive suggestion and see how far they'll come towards accepting it.

◇ Stay calm. Keep the emotional temperature down, even if the other person starts to get excited or angry. This shows that you are the one who's in control, even if they're an adult.

◇ Be prepared to negotiate and compromise.

Problems With Parents

Puberty is pretty tough on parents too. To you it may seem like all they want to do is nag or moan, but usually there's real worry and confusion behind their complaints. You are growing up and learning to be your own person, an individual. They are used to dealing with a little boy and, however obvious the signs have been that you're no longer exactly *little*, they've probably tried to pretend to themselves that everything is still the same. But it isn't. You have your own ideas and ambitions plus you probably want to spend a lot more time apart from them. Parents have to make the big adjustment of being less in control and much more trusting. It isn't easy! They want to protect you and keep you safe, and every time they read a headline about teenage violence, crime, alcoholism or drug taking, etc., they start to panic because they don't know exactly where you are or what you're doing every minute of the day. Try to remember that your mum and dad had their own experiences of growing up, so, even if they seem dead boring and straight now, they know all about the risks and temptations.

I don't think I even have a relationship with my parents! That's due to them being on a different planet. The only way I can cope is to walk away – they annoy me so much.

Chris, 15

My biggest rows were with my father, mainly because he suddenly wanted to take control of my studying and coursework and kept on about my savings. I didn't welcome this but at the same time I started to learn how they think and what influences them. I tend just to keep out of their affairs now, but it's still hard not to get annoyed and upset at some of their decisions or points of view.

Tony, 21

I've grown apart from mine. They don't seem as easy to talk to and they're always on at me about having to do jobs or be in at a certain time. I get annoyed, but I do try to reason with them. There's no other way.

Cleeton, 16

My parents are pretty cool – but they're divorced, and when I was about 14, I was aware of how keen my step-mum was on trying to point out my mother's bad points. This made me take everything she said with a pinch of salt because I know how hard a time my mum has had. Needless to say this caused rows with my step-mum and dad.

Daniel, 16

The good news is that this phase does pass, but it can take several years. If you're the oldest or only child it can be particularly hard as younger brothers often easily gain the trust and freedom that their older brothers have had to fight hard for.

Sex on the Brain

Suddenly everything seems to be about sex. You can't turn on the TV without seeing couples getting down to it, newspapers and magazines are full of half-naked bodies, and you're hyper-sensitive to everything anyone says, in case it has a double meaning. Many boys think about sex obsessively at this age – and some never grow out of it! You wonder what it will be like and long to try it, but there's also a lot of embarrassment and worry attached to the subject.

Parents can be particularly difficult. Helpful remarks about your 'love life', or aunts asking you whether you've 'got a girlfriend yet' make you want to crawl under the sofa and die. And sitting on the sofa with your parents while watching a love scene on TV is excruciating.

It may also feel as though your body is on show to the

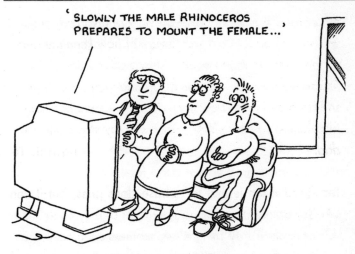

'SLOWLY THE MALE RHINOCEROS PREPARES TO MOUNT THE FEMALE...'

SEX ON THE BRAIN

whole world. Getting changed for games at school or being taken by your mum to buy some new clothes involves all sorts of pointed personal comments about your size and shape. Even your best mates can tease you and make you feel rotten. It can help to remember that they feel just as worried and embarrassed as you and teasing is often a defence mechanism to divert the heat from their own lack of self-confidence.

Am I Gay?

When you are growing up it's common to wonder whether you might be gay (homosexual). This means someone who is sexually attracted to their own sex. This can cause you a lot of secret anxiety – particularly if you hear other boys make crude jokes about homosexuality or use the term *gay* as a form of abuse. Your feelings could

67

be caused by having a crush on an older boy, feeling excited at the sight of naked bodies in the changing room or teasing by friends because you haven't got a girlfriend.

We don't know what makes people gay, but, although many religions and cultures consider it taboo, we now know there's nothing that can be done about it. You don't choose which sex you are attracted to – and pretending or suppressing your natural feelings means living a lie, and often leads to deep unhappiness. In other words, being gay is absolutely OK – but some boys think they are gay for the wrong reasons.

Having a crush or feeling attracted to an older person of the same sex is a common part of growing up. You're looking for role models and you might choose an older boy, a teacher at school, or someone famous whom you're never likely to meet. It's also a normal part of puberty to feel excited by the sight of naked bodies. Your brain is super-sensitive to anything associated with sex and you're interested in how other boys' bodies work as well as your own. And because your whole body is swamped with sex hormones making you feel charged up and frustrated, it can be easy to get into playful sex games with other boys.

None of these things necessarily means that you are gay, although you'll probably know whether you are or not by the time you're 14 or 15. In the meantime it's important not to feel pressurised into relationships with either sex before you feel ready for them. This is where talking to a trusted friend or adult or using a helpline can be so valuable. For more information see Chapter 9.

I sometimes worry that I ought to be gay. I have all the symptoms – I wear 'camp' clothes, I got a GCSE Grade A in Textiles, I loathe football but am into massage, aromatherapy and Japanese kitsch – but I definitely fancy girls, not men! It just shows that you shouldn't believe in stereotypes.   Daniel, 16

There was always a lot of touching and stuff at school. It was just all these urges flying around. None of us saw it as homosexual and I don't suppose many of the other boys actually were gay. However, I knew I definitely was by the time I was 14.   Jules, 23

I couldn't talk to my friends about being gay. The one person who helped me was an older woman who'd originally had a sexual interest in me. When I told her she helped me through the very difficult times of coming to terms with being gay and coping with the non-support of my immediate family.   Stephen, 20

If you think you're gay – or if there's anything you're really worried about – what you really want is a good friend. Friends see the real you. You can talk things through with them and they go away and think it over, then come back again and you haven't lost any face. You know you're lucky when you know you've got friends like that.   David, 24

How Many People Are Gay?

It's almost impossible to give an exact figure, because there's no obvious way to tell. However, recent surveys suggest the following:

◇ Between 1% and 3% of men are probably exclusively homosexual, i.e., only have sexual feelings for and relationships with other men.

◇ Around 2 or 3 times that number will have at least one experience of sex with another male in their lifetime.

◇ Many, many more will have had some form of sex play or mutual touching with another male at some time – usually when they're a child or teenager.

Self-Confidence

It's normal to feel extremely self-conscious at this age. Your body is changing and your moods may be swinging up and down. Perhaps you've got spots or feel worried because you're bigger or smaller than your friends. Everyone else seems to be self-assured and confident and you're convinced that secretly they all laugh at you. Of course the real secret is that everyone feels just the same way. However, some boys do suffer from more severe problems with self-confidence. Worries about blushing, asking a girl out and hearing her refuse, or even just putting your hand up to answer a question in class and getting the answer wrong, can all feel like massive problems.

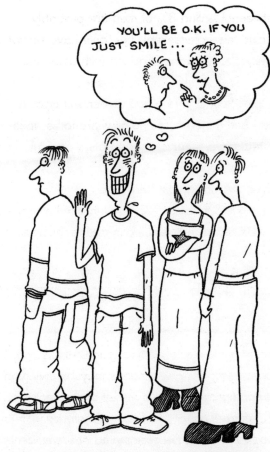

SELF-CONSCIOUSNESS/CONFIDENCE

The Cheat's Guide to Self-Confidence

The main trick to being confident is to *look* confident!
There are several ways to do this. The more you
practise them, the easier they become.

◇ Before you talk to someone for the first time or say
something in public you might feel scared and
jittery. Your heart probably beats faster and your
palms feel sweaty. This is the effect of adrenaline
rushing round your blood stream in response to
fear. But you can use it to help you focus. Take three
or four deep breaths, concentrating particularly on
exhaling (breathing out). This helps release tension
and slows down your heart rate.

◇ Say silently to yourself, 'I can do this, I can do this'.

◇ When you greet someone or want to make an
important point, look them in the eye. This can be

*The most worrying thing was relationships with girls at
school. I had no confidence in myself and never felt
popular. Asking a girl out that you really fancy was
always more awkward because the fear of rejection is
much greater.*   Tony, 21

difficult, so concentrate on trying to see what colour their eyes are. This gives the impression that you're looking deep into their eyes and makes you appear to be a genuine and confident person!

◇ Learn to ask open-ended questions to get a conversation going. This means anything that can't be answered with a simple yes or no. It puts the other person at ease and encourages them to talk. For example:

  ◇ How do you know John? (or whoever it is who's throwing the party)
  ◇ Which bands do you like?
  ◇ Why is it that we are the only people who don't seem to know anyone here?

◇ If you're interested in getting to know someone, ask them questions about themselves. It takes the pressure off you – and everyone loves a good listener.

Asking a girl out is still terrifying, but I've discovered that once you get talking it feels a lot better. If you've got something in common or something you can talk about to start off with, the whole thing is much easier.

Gareth, 20

If I could go back and give myself some advice, I'd say there are lots of things you're not going to understand in the slightest. Your emotions will run very hot and very cold. You'll be very unsure of yourself and self-conscious. It's difficult, but you've just got to remember that everyone goes through the same thing.   Geoff, 25

There are always people who look intimidating because they seem so self-confident, but actually they're bluffing and feel just as scared and insecure as you. But you only realise that later!   Paul, 18

When I was 13, I went to my first proper party and I was really nervous because I was very shy. My mum tried to be helpful and said I'd be OK if I just smiled at everyone there. I took her advice and ended up looking like a total moron! I know now that the important thing is just to be yourself.   Ed, 18

Depression

Puberty is an emotional roller coaster of ups and downs – but if there are more downs than ups, then you might need help. Depression isn't just feeling a bit miserable; it can also be a real illness needing professional help. It can creep up gradually, so that you don't realise what's happening and no one around you notices either. That's why it's so dangerous.

Symptoms of depression to look out for in yourself or your friends include:

◇ feeling sad and miserable
◇ feeling lonely
◇ feeling that nothing is worth bothering with
◇ wanting to stay in bed all the time
◇ having difficulty sleeping – either finding it hard to get off to sleep or waking up very early in the morning
◇ losing your appetite
◇ feeling that you are not worth much, or that no one would miss you if you were not around
◇ thinking about ways to harm yourself

Depressing Facts About Depression

◇ 1 in 3 young people in the UK feels depressed at least once a week.

◇ 7% of 13- to 18-year-olds report having suicidal thoughts.

◇ Depression increases the risk of alcohol or drug abuse.

◇ BUT drugs and alcohol can act as a further depressant and increase the risk of suicide.

Depression is a really serious problem for some boys. And it seems to be getting more common. Sometimes there's no obvious reason for it, but it can be associated with difficulties such as:

◇ worries about schoolwork or exams
◇ worries about friendships or girls
◇ problems at home, like parents arguing or splitting up, or constant rows about staying out late, etc.

Everyone thinks about suicide at some time, but then you come across people who are really serious. I once knew this guy who was definitely contemplating it. It freaked me out. He said the only reason he hadn't done it was because of his mum and how much it would hurt her. He really resented her for that. Johnny, 18

If I thought a friend of mine was going to kill themselves I'd definitely try to blow the whistle or prevent it, though they'd probably resent me interfering. But I know I'd be a bit selfish doing that, because it would be about me not wanting to lose a friend. Mark, 18

I definitely used to get depressed. My father is a chronic alcoholic and wife-beater. When I was 12, alone in the house, he returned from work drunk, crying about the state of his life and tried to kill himself in front of me. I had to call the ambulance. He put my mum in hospital on several occasions with his violence. Looking back, I don't know how we made it through. But I've never felt suicidal! There were lots of happy times too. Will, 22

I thought about killing myself once or twice, but it was mainly to do with questioning my sexuality. Luckily I found some other gay people who were older and who I could talk it over with.   Matt, 20

Depression – What to Do About It

If you start to feel depressed or notice that one of your friends is in a bad way, it's vital to get help immediately.

◇ First you need to talk about how you feel.
◇ If you don't want to talk to your family, you could try someone else, like a trusted teacher, the school nurse or counsellor, your best mate or their mum.
◇ You could also get help from your GP or a practice nurse or call a confidential helpline like the Samaritans or ChildLine where you can remain anonymous.

Even quite serious depression can usually be treated fairly quickly. Your own doctor should be able to help you or he may ask a specialist doctor to see you. Treatment might be with medicines or 'talking' therapies – often both are used together. For more information on how to go about getting help for depression and other problems see Chapter 9.

Problem Page

I'm 14 and the only one in my class who hasn't had sex. Everyone laughs at me and calls me gay. Does this mean I am gay?

You're in the best position to answer that! Do you feel more excited thinking about boys' bodies and being close to boys than you do about girls? If so, then you might be gay. If not, you probably aren't. But that doesn't alter the fact that a large proportion of your friends are either exaggerating or lying. Most young people are NOT having sex at the age of 14, but surveys repeatedly show that everyone thinks everyone else is doing it more than they really are. So it's tempting to exaggerate your own experience. This leads to lots of peer pressure and it's easy to end up lying about your love life or, even worse, having sex with someone you don't care about just to prove you can do it. Try to remember that the people who boast the loudest are often the most insecure.

DOC BOX
Suicide and Depression

◇ For some young people, depression gets so bad they try to kill themselves.
◇ Suicide is the second most common cause of death in older boys and young men in the UK. (The most common cause is road accidents.)
◇ 4 out of 5 young suicides are male.
◇ Although girls make more suicide attempts than boys, boys often use more violent methods and are therefore more likely to actually kill themselves.

My parents and relations keep making embarrassing comments like, 'How's your love life?' I hate it. What can I do?

It's toe-curlingly embarrassing, yet well-meaning adults still insist on asking this sort of thing. There's not much you can do about it at the time other than be rude, pro- voking a family row, or go into a major sulk. Much better to wait until later, then have a word with your mum or the offending relative and tell them straight that you hate it when people say things like that. Don't they remember how embarrassing it was when they were your age? This takes a bit of courage to do, but by talking straight, you're taking on the role of an equal, and you stand more chance of making your point.

I'm really worried I might be gay because when I was younger my friend and I used to touch each other and it felt good. We don't do it any more and we never talk about it. I think about sex a lot, but it's always with girls. But I'm scared I won't ever be able to do it because of what happened in the past.

Many, many boys have early same-sex experiences involving touching or masturbation. It's partly due to curiosity about your own body – comparing it to other people's and checking out whose works best. Even very young boys know that touching themselves feels good so having someone else do it can be even more exciting. But most boys grow out of this stage – although many, like you, feel guilty about what happened when they were younger. If your sexual fantasies are all about girls, then it sounds very unlikely that you are gay. But, even if you are, there's nothing wrong with being gay!

My best mate is cutting himself. I first realised when he kept wearing long sleeves in the summer, then one day I saw there were marks all over his wrists. At first I thought he'd tried to commit suicide, but he says it's just something he does when things get on top of him. This can't be safe and I'm really worried for him. But he's made me promise not to tell anyone.

Self-harm – which can include cutting, burning or stabbing yourself – is a serious problem for some young people but it often goes unrecognised. Your friend is probably telling you the truth when he says that he wasn't trying to kill himself, but any kind of self-harm is dangerous and it's a symptom of deep unhappiness and confusion. He needs help and he needs to talk to someone who understands what's going on. He may be too embarrassed or scared, but he's taken the first step by telling you. Unfortunately you can't handle this on your own. You must tell him that you're so worried you need to let an adult know. Hopefully he'll agree and choose to talk to someone himself, but if not, you must tell a teacher or the school nurse. I know your friend will be angry, but you could be saving his life. Some people who harm themselves do go on to attempt to commit suicide. Getting the right help early enough could prevent this.

Chapter 5

Body Maintenance

This chapter covers:
- ◇ Eating the right food
- ◇ Being overweight
- ◇ Being underweight
- ◇ Anorexia and eating disorders
- ◇ Smoking
- ◇ Alcohol and drugs
- ◇ Sleeping problems
- ◇ Exercise
- ◇ Keeping clean
- ◇ Shaving
- ◇ Spots and acne
- ◇ Music and hearing
- ◇ Headaches and migraines

Bodies are like cars – they work best if you can spare a bit of time to look after them. In this chapter you'll find some hints on how to stay fit and healthy.

Eating the Right Stuff

Food is fuel. Your body uses it for energy and breaks it down to use as building blocks for new growth of bone and muscle, and to replace old, dead cells. So there really is some truth in the saying 'you are what you eat'. It's particularly important to eat enough of the right kind of foods when you're growing up to help keep your body healthy and strong – but there's nothing very difficult about this.

To stay well you should try to eat something from each of the four major food groups every day:

◇ Protein: meat, fish, pulses (beans, lentils, etc.), milk and cheese
◇ Carbohydrate: cereals (bread, pasta, breakfast foods), rice, potatoes, etc.
◇ Fruit and Vegetables: choose ones you like – it doesn't have to be Brussels sprouts!
◇ Fat: butter, vegetable oils or dairy foods

Eating three meals a day including breakfast is particularly important. Breakfast is the one you're most likely to miss, because you're in a hurry or just don't feel like it. Even a bowl of cereal and milk can provide effective fuel to get your body going and contains lots of vitamins and minerals.

Being Overweight

Before a doctor or nurse decides if someone is overweight, they will check their height. People who are taller than average would be expected to weigh more than average.

Even if you feel you are overweight, don't try a crash

diet. They rarely work because you nearly always put all the weight back on again immediately afterwards. They can also be dangerous and, while you're still growing, too strict a diet could damage the way your bones and muscles form.

The best solution is to change your diet slightly. Eat more healthily and try to be sensible about what you do eat. Cut down on chocolate, crisps and snacks and fill up on pasta, baked potatoes and vegetables. At the same time try to take more exercise. Sitting in front of

DOC BOX

Risks Associated With Being Overweight

You need to be very overweight for at least 10 years for it to affect your health in the long-term.

If someone is 25% overweight for their height between the ages of 20 and 30, they are:

◇ 5 times more likely to die from diabetes
◇ 2.5 times more likely to die from a heart attack
◇ 1.5 times more likely to have a stroke

than someone who is average weight for their height.

Other medical problems that are associated with being overweight include:

the telly or computer burns hardly any calories. That's why one of the best ways to lose weight is to get more active. Even if you're not that keen on sport at school, try getting off the bus a stop earlier or taking the neighbour's dog for a walk. Don't try to lose weight – just keep to the same weight for several months while your height goes up. That way you'll start to look slimmer and you won't do yourself any harm. If you're still worried about your weight or shape talk to your school nurse or doctor. They'll be able to advise you on a

◇ feeling depressed
◇ breathlessness
◇ swollen ankles
◇ arthritis
◇ varicose veins
◇ hiatus hernias
◇ increased blood pressure
◇ increased blood fat levels
◇ kidney disease

But – remember that some other lifestyle choices can be as bad for your health as being overweight! People who smoke more than 25 cigarettes a day are 25 times more likely to die of lung cancer than non-smokers and twice as likely to die of heart disease.

healthy diet and give you an idea of what sort of weight and size you should be aiming for.

All my family's big – not surprising because we all eat a lot! I used to get teased at school because I couldn't run very fast and I'd go red and get out of breath quickly. And I got sore red patches where my thighs rubbed together. School games lessons were a nightmare so I learned to avoid them as much as possible. At 16, I left school (partly because of the bullying) and went to Sixth Form college. Maybe I was just happier, or perhaps because I had a long walk to and from the station, I started to lose weight. And I felt better. I met new friends and started going out at weekends and the weight just continued to drop off. At first I thought it was some kind of magic then I realised that the rest of my family was still sitting on the sofa watching TV and stuffing their faces. That's why they were all overweight. I realised I didn't have to be like that, though it's still hard when Mum tries to 'feed me up'!   Chris, 19

Being Underweight

Many boys are self-conscious about being too thin. This is a common phase when you start growing fast and your body stretches out. It can take a while for muscle development to catch up and for your shoulders and chest to fill out. Mothers are notorious for worrying that their beloved boys are too skinny and often ask their family doctor for help. The doctor or nurse will certainly check your weight and height to make sure that it's roughly right for your age, but as long as you are eating well, there's usually nothing to worry about.

I know mums nag, but mine went on all the time about me not eating. At 15, I'd grown fast and I was a bit of a beanpole. And often I didn't feel like meals, especially not if it meant sitting down listening to everyone going on at me. Mum always tried to make me eat 'properly' and it became a real battle. She made out I was doing it deliberately to upset her but she never understood that I'd eat when I was hungry and wouldn't if I wasn't. Simple as that! I did eat lots of junk food – crisps and stuff. But I also drank lots of milk – usually late at night. Another thing for her to moan about. Jake, 17

Eating Disorders

Sometimes being underweight *is* a problem. Eating disorders are illnesses where food – eating or not eating it – becomes an obsession which interferes with normal life and health. The best known eating disorder is *anorexia nervosa*. This is a serious condition that can affect both sexes – though it's more common in girls. It usually begins when someone feels self-conscious about their size and starts to diet. However, often they think they're much fatter than they really are and this perception continues even as they lose weight. About 1 in every 100 teenage girls and 1 in every 2,000 boys are affected by anorexia. They get thinner and thinner and don't believe their friends and

87

family when they tell them that they're already thin enough. Anorexia is often associated with depression, being scared of losing control, stress or a fear of getting fat.

Other effects of anorexia include:

◇ dry skin
◇ increased fine body hair

Case History

Joe had always been a bit plump and his mates teased him about it. He had quite bad asthma as a child and he had to have steroid tablets several times each year. These made him feel really hungry. When he was 14 he suddenly got very miserable about his weight and began to diet. He felt starving hungry all the time, but was delighted with the way he was losing weight – around 1 kg (2 lbs) every week.
He didn't really know how to diet healthily – he just stopped having breakfast, had a couple of apples for lunch and then picked at his dinner at home. At first his mum was pleased he was dieting but when he got down to the right weight for his height Joe just didn't seem to be able to stop the diet. He felt hungry, but at the same time he felt really in control of something for the first time in his life. He quite liked the fact that his mum's friends stopped him when they saw him and asked if he was all right as he looked so pale. He began to run early each morning and soon he was up

- ◇ slowing of heart rate
- ◇ difficulty sleeping
- ◇ poor concentration
- ◇ constipation
- ◇ constantly feeling cold
- ◇ osteoporosis (weakening of the bones)

to 7 km a day. That way he could eat just a little bit more and still lose weight. But he felt freezing cold most of the time and often felt faint.

Eventually his mum was so worried that she tried to persuade Joe to see a doctor, but Joe got really angry and said there wasn't a problem and people should just leave him alone. It wasn't until he saw some holiday photos that he realised just how ill he looked – he was down to 51 kg which was very light for someone of his height (173 cm). He realised there were lots of things worrying him and that he'd been concentrating on losing weight instead of thinking about all the other issues. He agreed to go and see his GP and, after talking with him, admitted that he had become anorexic. He was referred to a specialist in eating disorders in boys and took part in group therapy sessions. He was horrified to find out that 1 in every 5 people who have anorexia die from it. It took several months for Joe to feel back in control of his eating and his weight and, even now – three years later – he finds that he thinks about food all the time.

Another eating disorder is binge eating, where a person sometimes eats normally but other times can't seem to stop themselves eating everything in sight. *Bulimia* is an illness which combines binge eating with strict dieting. Bulimics usually make themselves sick to get rid of the food they feel so guilty about eating. This problem is difficult for families and friends to spot as the sufferer often manages to stay a normal weight for their height. But, like anorexia, it can be very dangerous. It can cause a low potassium level in the blood, leading to sudden collapse and sometimes death.

DOC BOX
WARNING

Anorexia can kill. By starving your body you can alter its chemical balance leading to heart failure or dehydration. Even for those people who do get better, recovery can be very slow.

If you are worried about whether you or someone you know has this problem, you must get help as soon as possible. If you feel you can't talk to your parents about it, speak to your GP, a practice nurse or your school nurse. For more information on where to get help see Chapter 9.

Smoking

Smoking is definitely bad for your health, yet 1 in 3 boys aged 15 to 16 admit to being regular smokers – although the number is now starting to fall.

Every year in the UK, 120,000 people die from smoking-related diseases. This compares to 5,000 people killed every year in road accidents. The younger you start smoking, the more dangerous it is – starting with an increased risk of coughs, colds and chest infections, leading to much more serious diseases that can kill, like cancer and heart disease.

Most young people start smoking because they see older people doing it and they want to look cool – or their friends all smoke and they don't want to feel left out. It can easily become a nervous habit, giving you something to do with your hands when you feel unsure of yourself. But nicotine, the chemical in tobacco, is highly addictive and, for many, those first few cigarettes are the start of a life-long, love-hate relationship with tobacco.

Luckily there is help around to break the addiction. Some people use nicotine substitutes like patches or gum, but the most important thing is to decide you don't want to be a smoker any more. For information websites and support groups see Chapter 9.

Alcohol and Drugs

If alcohol was invented today, there is no way that it would be legal! Long-term health problems and deaths from alcohol-related diseases are on the increase and young people drink more heavily now than ever before.

Drugs of all kinds seem to be increasingly common. Most teenagers will have been offered them or will know people who have used them – assuming they haven't experimented themselves. But, just because there are drugs around, it doesn't mean they are safe. The very fact that they are illegal means there are no quality controls and you can never be sure what you are buying – and risking.

Alcohol and drugs – whether legal or illegal – have one important thing in common. People take them because they make them feel good – by altering their mood and how they see the world. Whether they get you high like E or acid, or bring you down like alcohol or sedative drugs, they affect your judgement. This means you're more likely to make poor decisions, take risks or have an accident. For example:

⬦ The majority of road accidents which result in the death or serious injury of a young person involve alcohol.
⬦ Alcohol and many drugs act as depressants and there's a strong link between their abuse and suicide in young people.
⬦ Young people who have sex when they've been drinking alcohol are less likely to use protection and are more at risk of unwanted pregnancy and sexually transmitted infection. Many young people who have

sex for the first time when they are drunk regret it later.

◇ The majority of violent incidents and street crimes are due to the effects of alcohol or a desire to raise money for drugs.

Sleep

When you're younger, you do most of your growing while you're asleep! So sleep is important for growth, but you probably already know that not having enough sleep affects you in other ways too. Apart from leaving you feeling tired and short-tempered, lack of sleep interferes with your concentration and performance so you'll find it much harder to focus at school. Some people also find that lack of sleep makes them more likely to catch any colds or bugs that are going round.

Everyone's different, but between the ages of about 8 and 18, eight hours' sleep a night is considered ideal. Many teenagers have no trouble sleeping – it's just that they prefer to go to bed late and sleep in later in the morning! Unfortunately this often doesn't fit in with school life. The occasional late night is fine, but it's much better for you to try to keep to a regular pattern of sleep. That way you'll find it easier to fall asleep when you do go to bed, rather than tossing and turning until the early hours of the morning.

Insomnia

Insomnia is the inability to sleep and it's common to experience short periods of it while you're growing up. Sometimes it's caused by worry, for example about school, exams, family problems or even that you're not getting enough sleep. If you find you have problems getting off to sleep at night, try the following:

◇ Develop a good bedtime routine.
◇ Avoid coffee, tea, cola and chocolate after six o'clock, as these are all stimulants that can keep you buzzing.
◇ Avoid playing computer games last thing at night – these can also over-stimulate your mind.
◇ A nice warm bath and some relaxing music can help you unwind.
◇ Make sure your room is dark enough – in the summer you might need to drape an old, dark-coloured towel over your window if your curtains let in too much light.
◇ Try not to panic if you can't nod off straight away – just being in bed is restful. But if you find yourself lying there for ages unable to sleep it's better to get up, make yourself a warm, caffeine-free drink and walk around or read a book for 20 minutes rather than lie in bed and worry about it.

Most people can get into a good sleep routine by following these tips, but if you still find yourself lying awake worrying or are waking early in the morning and generally feeling low, you could be suffering from stress or depression. It might be a good idea to go and talk to your GP.

DOC BOX
Sleeping Pills

Although sleeping pills may seem to offer an easy answer to insomnia they are rarely a good idea. They may help you sleep at first but you quickly become used to them and they don't do anything to help you develop good sleeping habits. Some brands of sleeping pills and medicines are now sold over the counter in pharmacies. These usually contain antihistamines which have the side effect of making you feel drowsy and confused. Often the effects last into the next day so, although you may have slept, you still find it hard to concentrate. If you really think you need sleeping pills it's best to talk to your GP first.

Sport and Exercise

Exercise is important to keep you fit and healthy – not just now, but in later life too. And people who get into the habit of exercising when they're at school tend to keep it up when they are adults. This can dramatically reduce their risk of dying from illnesses like heart disease, strokes and diabetes.

Besides helping to get your body toned and in good shape, exercise has an added bonus. It releases chemicals called endorphins which make you feel a bit high. Like dieting, exercise can sometimes become addictive so it's important you don't let it start to rule your life. And, while running a marathon might seem like a good idea, most doctors wouldn't recommend it until you are 18. Too much running can cause damage to growing bones.

DOC BOX
Choose a Sport You Like, Then Do It

Not everyone enjoys school-organised sports, so it's important to find something you do like. This could be anything from traditional sports like football, swimming and rugby, to dancing, skateboarding or rollerblading. Ideally you should exercise for 5 sessions of 30 minutes each per week. The important thing is that you should feel a bit breathless but not so shattered that you can't speak! It's better to do 'little and often' rather than no exercise for weeks and then go mad.

Keeping Clean

During puberty your sweat changes and becomes much stronger and that's why so many teenage boys smell! But by keeping yourself and your clothes clean you can reduce the problem a lot. Fresh sweat isn't too bad, but as it dries and goes stale it becomes unpleasant – whether it's on you or on your clothes.

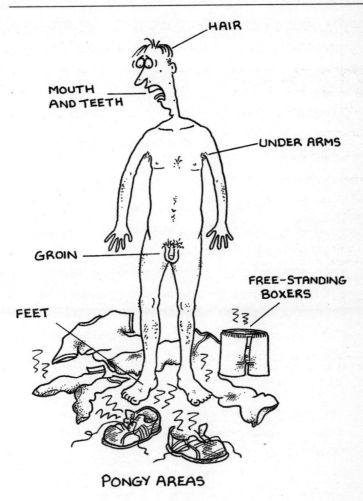

HAIR

MOUTH AND TEETH

UNDER ARMS

GROIN

FREE-STANDING BOXERS

FEET

PONGY AREAS

To avoid smelling, you need to shower or bath every day. This means rubbing soap or shower gel all over – not just standing under the water for a few minutes! Don't forget to wash your penis and testicles too – pulling your foreskin back to get rid of any cheesy-smelling smegma. For more details and tips see Chapter 6. Most boys over 12 need

97

Antiperspirants and Deodorants

Antiperspirants can help cut down on the amount of sweat you produce, while deodorants help cut out the smell. Both come as sticks, roll-ons or sprays. Some products contain both and many have their own strong smell, so you need to try several to find one that works best for you.

But no amount of deodorant or perfume can disguise smelly bodies and clothes, so you need to get clean – and keep clean

Some people do sweat more than others and there are special creams and sprays available from pharmacists to help with this. You need to ask at the pharmacy counter because they won't be on display in the main shop.

clean underwear every day – especially socks. And don't forget that you often sweat in bed, so try to change your sheets at least once a week too.

I don't reckon boys really notice that they smell. It's normal and healthy and there's nothing wrong with sweat. But I've got one friend who really has a problem. It's OK most of the time, but if we end up crashing for the night at someone's house you really don't want to be in the same room with him when he takes his shoes off. The stink is unbelievable. Matthew, 16

Mouth and Teeth

The chances are you have healthier teeth than your parents did at your age. This is mainly due to the addition of fluoride to the water when you were growing up. But that doesn't mean you should neglect your teeth – or your dentist! Every time you eat something, particularly if it's sweet or sticky, a residue is left on your teeth, attracting bacteria that gradually attack the teeth and gums. Brushing your teeth regularly – at least twice a day – is the best defence against this. When brushing it's important to get to all the bits you can't see, i.e., behind the teeth and around the back. You should see your dentist every six to twelve months and they'll tell you whether or not you're doing a good job.

Bad breath (medical name *halitosis*) can be a major turn-off in even the best relationship. It's often caused by poor mouth hygiene – though anxiety, dehydration, hunger or the after-effects of too much beer or curry play their part as well. It's very hard to tell whether your own breath smells. Blowing into your cupped hands and sniffing doesn't really work. Your best bet is to ask someone you trust, like your mum or your dentist. They should give you an honest answer. A quick solution is to use a mouthwash, breath spray or suck some mints, but developing a better brushing technique and asking your dentist for advice about preventing or treating possible gum disease are the long-term cures. Dentists also recommend brushing your tongue (this feels very strange at first) to help remove some of the pong-producing bacteria.

My mum always nagged me about cleaning my teeth but there never seemed much point. It didn't make any difference when I went to the dentist because I never had to have anything done. Then there was this girl I really liked but when I finally managed to kiss her she sort of pulled away and wrinkled her nose. Later I heard she'd told her friends I had dog breath. Since then I've brushed my teeth regularly! Max, 17

Shaving

For many boys, starting to shave is one of the biggest steps towards growing up. You're probably already aware which of your friends need to shave and which don't, and you might feel left out if you're one of the later developers. People with darker skin and hair tend to have earlier beard growth, but even for them, the first hairs are usually soft and fine – not thick enough to grow a real beard or moustache. Shaving is a personal choice

DOC BOX
Athlete's Foot

This is a common and uncomfortable condition – which doesn't only happen to athletes! It's caused by a tiny fungus that lives between your toes and likes hot, sweaty feet. Wearing trainers and tight nylon socks makes it worse. You get patches of sore, red

– both *whether* you do it and *how* you do it. There's no medical reason to shave, but many schools insist that pupils are clean-shaven.

I'd realised I had ugly bum-fluff developing but didn't know what to do about it. Luckily my parents had noticed too so they gave me an electric shaver for my 14th birthday! I taught myself . . . but I've improved a lot since. Tom, 18

My dad kept telling me that I didn't need to shave, even though I was getting a lot of growth on my face and people were going on about it at school. Eventually I wore him down and he showed me how to do it by using an electric shaver on one side of my face. I think most people just use what their dad uses or what they've been given for Christmas. One guy got given nose clippers which he was really offended about! Cyrus, 18

skin which often flakes off and it's very, very itchy.

You can get powder or sprays for athlete's foot from the pharmacist and this usually helps a lot. But, to stop it coming back, you need to make sure that you change your socks every day, always dry carefully between your toes after a bath or shower and air your feet by walking about without shoes or socks as often as possible.

My dad had a 'serious' talk to me about shaving. I'd already watched him doing it so I started with an electric razor, an old-fashioned type, but it made my skin very sore. If I had a lot of spots I couldn't shave when I needed or wanted to. Also I hated the smell in the shaver as it takes on all the gunk and smell of the skin. After a year or so I switched to wet shaving which was a bit of a hassle but felt much cleaner.   Kevin, 24

If you haven't already had a lesson from your family expert, try the following tips:

◇ For best results use a wet-shave razor.
◇ To soften the skin, either shave after you've had a bath or shower or pre-wash your skin with warm water.
◇ Lather your face with shaving foam or gel – but don't use too much. Try different types to find the one that suits you best.
◇ Be sure the razor you're using is sharp. You're more likely to damage your skin with older, blunt blades.
◇ Move the razor across your skin in the same direction the hair grows. This reduces friction and irritation.
◇ Rinse the razor several times as you shave to keep the blade clean and efficient.
◇ Rinse your face with warm water when you've finished.

Choosing a Razor or Shaver

The two main choices are wet-shave razors or electric shavers.

A wet-shave razor can be disposable plastic with a metal blade, or more solid, usually metal with replaceable razor blades. Electric shavers range from fairly cheap and simple to very expensive and complicated.

In practice, most boys use whatever they see their father use, or the electric shaver they are given for Christmas or a birthday.

Electric shavers are quick and easy to use, but can be harsh on the skin as you use them dry.

Wet-shaving is slower and more fiddly but gives a closer shave and usually causes less irritation to the skin.

◇ Small cuts and nicks are common when you start or if you're shaving in a hurry.
◇ Use your own razor and don't share it with family or friends as it could spread an infection.

Spots

All over your skin (but particularly on your face) there are tiny glands called *sebaceous* glands. These produce an oily substance called *sebum* which 'waterproofs' your skin. During puberty the male hormones (mainly testosterone) make you produce more sebum so your skin looks and feels greasy. Often the sebaceous glands get blocked by plugs of sebum and this causes them to swell up into whiteheads or pimples. As the plug of sebum is exposed to the air it turns black, making a blackhead.

Acne

Many teenagers develop lots of spots – not only on their face, but also on their back, shoulders and chest. This is acne. Coping with it isn't always easy but try dealing with it like this:

◇ Keep your skin as clean as possible by using a medicated soap or lotion that you can buy from the supermarket or pharmacy.

◇ Use spot creams to help dry the spots out.

◇ Get some fresh air every day (and some sunshine if possible) as this also helps dry the skin a bit.

◇ If this doesn't work, talk to the pharmacist at the prescriptions counter as they can give you stronger creams and lotions.

◇ If these haven't worked after 3 or 4 weeks go and talk to your GP. He/she can prescribe special ointments or pills to zap the acne – though you'll have to use them for 4 to 6 weeks to see a real difference.

◇ In the rare cases where acne is still a problem, your doctor can arrange for you to see a

dermatologist (special skin doctor) for more
treatment.

DOC BOX
Spots

Everyone has bacteria living on their skin. These bugs
can get into the blocked glands causing an infection.
The bacteria keep reproducing and white blood cells
gather to try to fight them off. This causes:

◇ swelling
◇ redness
◇ sometimes quite a lot of pain

Eventually the pressure inside the spot gets too great
and it bursts – like a volcano – and the swelling
and pain ease off. Everyone is tempted to squeeze
their spots, but by doing so you risk transferring
more bugs from dirty fingers or fingernails and
pushing the infection deeper down into your skin,
causing a worse problem. However, if you must
squeeze, make sure your hands and skin are really
clean and then cover your fingers in a clean tissue.

Headaches

Most people suffer from occasional headaches. It can be
useful to work out if there's anything causing them. For

example, stress affects people in different ways so if you are struggling to meet homework deadlines or are anxious about a relationship, it could make you very tense. When this happens all the muscles of the body can

DOC BOX
Migraine Headaches

What are they?

A migraine is a type of headache which often starts with a pain on one side of the head and can last from 4 to 72 hours. Some people have migraine headaches several times a month, others only once or twice a year. They usually feel very sick or even vomit with them. Many people need to lie down in a dark room while they have a migraine attack.

Some sufferers get an odd warning (an aura) before the headache starts. Features of an aura include:

◇ dazzling/flashing lights
◇ black spots in front of the eyes
◇ weakness, numbness and/or tingling in face, hand, arm or leg
◇ problems seeing or speaking normally
◇ feeling very depressed, irritable, drowsy or thirsty

tighten up and, as the neck muscles get tense, pain moves up from the muscles at the base of the head and neck to the front of the head. This can be felt as a throbbing pain – a tension headache. It usually only lasts for a short while

What causes migraines?

Experts aren't sure. It might be due to changes in blood flow in the brain or in the level of a nerve transmitter. These are usually triggered by something else – anything from an allergy (often to food, coffee or alcohol) to stress, to glare from the sun, a change in sleep pattern or missing a meal. If your parents have migraines it's much more likely that you will get them too.

Treatment (With any medication, always read the label carefully.) If mild painkillers like Paracetomol and Ibuprofen don't work for you, talk to your doctor as he/she can prescribe preventive treatments.

Try to pinpoint and reduce whatever it is that causes the migraines:

◇ Avoid known 'problem' foods, such as coffee, chocolate, cheese, red wine.
◇ Avoid too much alcohol.
◇ Deal with stress at an early stage, for example, by doing more exercise or learning relaxation techniques.

– perhaps a few hours – and it doesn't make you feel sick. Simple painkillers can help, but it's a good idea to try to find out why the tension is happening and deal with that if you can, rather than keep resorting to painkillers.

Music and Loss of Hearing

Loud music can damage your hearing – but most young people don't think it will happen to them. In one survey,

---

DOC BOX
Personal Stereos – Health Warning

Personal stereos are a particular problem as they are often turned up very loud to allow people to listen to music when there is lots of background noise. In a quiet room, most people can hear the music well through headphones when it is at a level of about 60 decibels. In a busy street, they usually turn the volume up to over 80 decibels.

If a personal stereo is used during exercise the problem is made even worse. When you are exercising, your body diverts blood to the muscles in your arms and legs. There's less blood flow to the ears and this makes the cells responsible for hearing particularly vulnerable to damage.

Doctors say that if you want to listen to music while you exercise, you should have the volume no higher than halfway – and you should only listen for 30 minutes maximum.

---

8 out of 10 clubbers were not worried about their hearing – but 6 out of 10 people who go to clubs regularly, and 7 out of 10 concert-goers do have problems with hearing afterwards – and in some cases this can be permanent!

The sounds produced at concerts and clubs can be as loud as 120 decibels. That is louder than a pneumatic drill. By law, workers using noisy equipment have to be protected from sounds louder than 85 decibels.

Problem Page

I have problems with spots and my mum says it's because I eat too much chocolate. Is this true?

Over-indulging in sweets and chocolate isn't particularly good for you but doesn't cause spots or acne. Most teenagers suffer from spots at times but if you've always got more than 2 or 3 on the go it's worth taking some preventive action. Look at the section on spots and start with the washes and creams that you can buy from a pharmacist. If that doesn't do the trick, ask a pharmacist or doctor for further help.

I've always been quite chunky and I'm not very good at sport. People make fun of me at school and call me names. I'd like to be thinner but everyone in my family is big. Does that mean there's nothing I can do about it?

It means it's harder for you to do anything about it. Your height and general shape, particularly shoulder and hip width, are inherited from your parents. The tendency to be overweight also runs in families, but a lot of that is due to eating habits and patterns. Presumably your mum or someone at home prepares your main meals. Some families just get into the habit of eating too much! If you really think you're overweight for your height have a word with your mum or whoever is in charge of the kitchen at home and ask if they can help you eat more healthily. You don't necessarily have to eat less or go hungry, just eat more rice, pasta, potatoes and fruit and vegetables and steer clear of sweet and greasy things. Do the same at school and make a point of not choosing chips or crisps or sticky puddings for lunch. And cut down on snacks of crisps and sweets. Eat some fruit or a low-fat yoghurt if you're hungry between meals. If you do this and try to take some extra exercise, you'll soon find that your body shape starts to change. Remember you may not lose weight but, if you're still growing, you'll start to look slimmer.

My mum's always on at me to eat more fruit and vegetables but I hate green stuff! Do I really need it?

Experts recommend that you should have at least 5 helpings of fruit and vegetables a day to help you grow properly and stay healthy. It's a good idea to vary these but there's no point trying to force down something you hate. Steamed and baked potatoes contain lots of vitamins (especially in the skin) and carrots, bananas and many other vegetables and fruit, including salad leaves and frozen vegetables are also excellent sources of vitamins and minerals. One glass of fruit juice, such as orange or pineapple, contains all the vitamin C you need for one day – but try to stick to real fruit juices *without* added sugar, sweeteners, etc.

After I've been to a gig or concert I sometimes get a crackling, buzzing noise in my ears. My mum says I'm damaging my hearing with loud music, but it always goes away again. This isn't dangerous is it?

Loud noises – at clubs and concerts, for example, often cause *tinnitus* – ringing in the ears. Sometimes this only lasts for a few hours, but it can be permanent – and the damage builds up – so if you go to lots of concerts, the problem could get worse and worse. It's caused when the tiny cells inside your ears which are responsible for hearing become over-stimulated by loud noises. In severe cases they are killed off altogether, resulting in permanent hearing loss. The ability to hear high-pitched noises usually goes first. More and more DJs now wear earplugs when they are working. Maybe you should think about protecting your ears too!

I've been smoking for about a year – only about 10 to 15 a day – but it's affecting how well I can run and play sport. I thought it would be easy to give up, but it isn't. I

111

know smoking is bad for you and have already probably damaged my body, so is it too late to do anything about it?

Definitely not! It can be very hard to break the habit of smoking, but the longer you leave it the harder it will be. You've got a good reason to want to quit so ring one of the helplines in Chapter 9 and get advice from the experts. The good news is that once you stop smoking your body starts to repair the damage it caused, reducing the risk of all those smoking-related diseases.

Chapter 6

Looking After Your Willy

This chapter covers:
- ◇ General hygiene
- ◇ Tight foreskin
- ◇ Problems with your penis
- ◇ Problems with your testes

This chapter is about how to look after that all-important piece of tackle that hangs between your legs. This includes general hygiene (keeping it clean) as well as common worries and problems which can affect the health of your penis and testes.

General Hygiene – Keeping Your Willy Clean

Two things can cause your penis to become smelly and unpleasant. Because you urinate (pee) several times a day there will be a build-up of dried, stale urine around the end of your penis. You may also notice a white, cheesy discharge called *smegma* which collects under the foreskin and, if not washed off carefully, turns rancid and smelly.

Try the following tips for keeping your penis clean and healthy:

◇ When you urinate or pee slide your foreskin back first so that urine doesn't collect on the inside of it.

◇ Have a bath or shower every day and slide your foreskin back towards the base of your penis so you can wash carefully underneath it and round the head.

◇ Afterwards dry the end of your penis and the foreskin carefully.

◇ Then pull the foreskin back down over the head again.

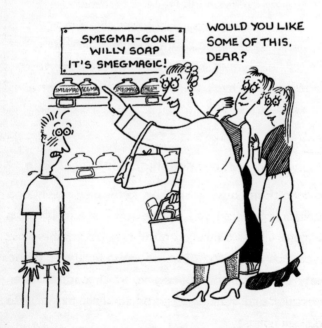

DOC BOX
Signs to Watch Out for in Your Penis

You should ask you doctor for advice if you notice any of the following:

◇ discharge or pus from your penis
◇ difficulty or discomfort on pulling back the foreskin
◇ needing to pee frequently with stinging sensation when you do
◇ blood in semen at ejaculation
◇ foreskin becomes too tight to push back down over the head of the penis after an erection, causing redness, swelling and pain. **This is a medical emergency (para-phimosis); see your doctor or visit a hospital A&E department as soon as possible.**

Possible Problems With Your Penis

Spots on the penis

Although it can be a bit alarming to discover spots on your penis they're as likely to grow there as anywhere else on your body. They are rarely serious and often just a side-effect of your penis living in warm, moist conditions, i.e., tucked inside your pants, where bacteria can multiply and spots can flourish.

Symptoms The most common type of spots are small white pimples which often appear on the underside of the penis

115

or under the foreskin around the head or glans.

Treatment They usually go away on their own as long as you keep yourself clean with regular washing using a mild soap. Don't pick or squeeze them in case they become infected.

DOC BOX
Tight Foreskin

Some boys find it very difficult to pull their foreskin back from the end of their penis, usually because the foreskin is too tight. Sometimes it's possible to stretch it gently by using soap and water in the shower and pulling a little further every day. However you should NEVER force it. If gentle pulling or rubbing doesn't work or if there's any discomfort, it's important to check with a doctor.

You could need to be circumcised or the doctor might just arrange for you to have a small snip in the end of your foreskin to loosen it. Both of these are minor operations which would be done in hospital under an anaesthetic.

Balanitis

This is a common problem caused by bacteria, which are naturally present on the skin of the penis, growing out of control. It's more common in men who are not circumcised because the foreskin keeps the skin under it warm and moist, encouraging the bacteria to grow. You are more likely to get it if you have diabetes.

Symptoms Balanitis is an inflammation of the head of the penis causing a blotchy rash or general redness – sometimes with a discharge. Your penis may be hot, itchy or uncomfortable, or, in spite of looking different, feel completely normal.

Treatment This condition is NOT sexually transmitted but can be linked with poor hygiene, i.e., not washing every day. Medication is rarely necessary – the important thing is to keep the skin under the foreskin clean and dry. Washing more carefully and more regularly will usually clear up the symptoms and prevent further problems. If you do get repeated attacks of balanitis and regular washing isn't making any difference, you should see your doctor.

Para-phimosis

This is an extremely painful condition where the foreskin (often tight to begin with) cannot be drawn back down to cover the head of the penis after an erection.

Symptoms Following masturbation or sex the foreskin appears to tighten around the base of the head of the penis looking (and feeling!) like a ring of swollen skin. As it cuts off the flow of blood the head or glans becomes increasingly swollen and painful.

Treatment You may be able to gently push the foreskin down yourself. It can take a while but if you feel you're making progress, carry on with it. However, if it won't budge you need to contact a doctor or hospital A&E

department urgently. The longer you leave it the worse it will get. A doctor may use a local anaesthetic cream to numb the foreskin and the head of the penis while he/she draws it back down again, or you may need to have an operation to loosen the foreskin.

Urine infections

More common in girls than boys, these are caused by bacteria entering the urethra (urine passage) causing infections in the bladder or even further up in the kidneys.

Symptoms You may feel that you need to pee frequently and when you do it could sting. Urine infections can also cause backache or groin-ache, nausea or vomiting, and a high temperature.

Treatment Because urine infections can lead to permanent damage to the kidneys if left untreated, it's always important to see your doctor if you suspect you have one. They will listen to your symptoms and may ask you to give a sample of urine but are unlikely to examine you or do anything embarrassing. Most infections are easily cured with antibiotics.

Bleeding from the penis

Although this is uncommon it's obviously alarming and should always be reported to your doctor.

Symptoms Bleeding from the end of your penis or blood in your urine (sometimes just making it look smoky) or in your semen when you ejaculate. This could be caused by something quite simple like a burst blood vessel or could be a symptom of an internal disease like a severe kidney infection or kidney stones. You may also feel quite ill and have a high temperature.

Treatment Your doctor will want to listen to your symptoms and take a sample of urine to test. Most infections can be cleared up with a course of antibiotics but you may have to go for further tests.

Possible Problems With Your Testes

You probably already know that your testes (balls) are very, very sensitive and, if they get knocked or kicked, it

DOC BOX
Signs to Watch Out for in Your Testes

You should ask your doctor for advice if you notice any of these:

◇ a lump in one testicle
◇ pain or tenderness for no obvious reason
◇ pain after injury which does not wear off after one hour
◇ a swelling or build up of fluid inside your scrotum
◇ a heavy or dragging feeling in the groin or scrotum
◇ a gradual and definite increase in size of one testicle

119

can be agonising. Some problems in the testes happen very suddenly while others are slower growing, but potentially more dangerous. It's important to know what your own testes look and feel like and to be on the lookout for any change as an early warning sign of disease.

How to check your testicles
Just as girls and young women are taught to check their breasts for lumps and early warning signs of cancer, you should make sure you get to know your testicles by checking them regularly. The best time is in the bath or shower because warm water helps the skin of the scrotum to relax so any lumps or bumps can be felt more easily.

Cradle them in the palms of your hands and feel the difference in size. One is almost always larger and lying lower. That's normal, but you need to be on the lookout for any change from month to month.

Roll each testicle between your fingers and thumb to check for any bumps or swellings. They should be smooth, apart from along the top and back where the sperm duct leaves the testicle carrying the sperm to the penis.

Finally examine your scrotum by touch and in a mirror to check for any lumps or swellings under the skin.

Testicular cysts
Cysts are small pockets filled with fluid, making them feel like a hard lump. They're very common but cause a lot of anxiety in boys and men.

Symptoms A hard lump, usually on the upper side of one testis. It doesn't usually hurt, but does feel quite solid to the touch. A good tip is to shine a torch through the skin of your scrotum. The lump may glow, showing that it contains fluid and not solid matter. This is a good sign, **but it's best to check ALL lumps with your doctor.**

Treatment Most cysts go away on their own, but your GP can arrange for you to have an ultrasound test if necessary. This doesn't hurt, takes only a few minutes and can usually tell you and the doctor straight away what type of lump you're dealing with.

Testicular cancer

This is the most common cancer in young men. It's been on the increase in the UK for the last 20 years and there are now around 1,500 cases a year. It is the biggest single cause of cancer-related deaths in men aged 15 to 35.

Symptoms The first symptom of testicular cancer is a small, hard lump in the testis. However, the majority of lumps are NOT cancer but cysts (see previous page). The lump is usually painless, starting about the size of a pea, but, if left untreated, the whole testicle will gradually become swollen.

Treatment Testicular cancer has a very high cure rate (95%) if it's detected early enough. This is why it's so important to get to know the feel of your own testes and to check any change or lump out with your doctor. If you find a lump your doctor will arrange for an ultrasound scan. If it does prove to be cancer, treatment will be surgery plus perhaps radiotherapy and/or drugs. If left untreated testicular cancer can kill you!

Varicocoeles

These are swellings caused by varicose (swollen or enlarged) veins. A fairly common problem, which, if left untreated, could possibly decrease your fertility (ability to produce sperm).

Symptoms Swollen, darkish red lump (looks like a bag of worms) usually on the underside of the testes. It may be painless or cause a dull ache, but the swelling usually feels warm to the touch. It occurs more on the left side than the right.

Treatment See your doctor to have the swelling checked. It may be necessary to have a small operation to tie off the veins and reduce the swelling before it causes further problems.

Trauma

Being hit or kicked in the testicles is a nightmare for any boy or man. It's a common risk during sport, fights or general rough play, and even the thought of it is probably enough to make you want to cross your legs.

Although a blow to the testes can cause agonising pain and often make you feel nauseous or sick, most incidents are not dangerous. But it's important to know the warning signs for serious problems so you can call the doctor if necessary.

Symptoms Because your testicles hang outside your body, unprotected by bones or muscle, they are very vulnerable. If they're hit or kicked you will feel severe pain plus nausea, light-headedness, dizziness and sweating. You may fall to the ground on your knees or curl up in agony.

Treatment In most cases the pain and other symptoms should start to wear off in less than an hour. As with any other injury, putting a cold pack (or a towel-wrapped bag of frozen peas) on it can help reduce the pain and swelling. If the pain lasts longer than one hour – or if you suffer extreme swelling or discolouration of the testes or there's a puncture wound, you should see a doctor or go to a hospital A&E department as soon as possible. They will check for internal injury and bleeding.

Better Safe Than Sorry

Wearing a 'box' when playing sports where there's a high risk of injury may protect you from severe pain.

Testicular torsion

This is an occasional problem particularly in boys between the ages of about 12 and 18. Inside the scrotum the testicles are secured at either end, but one can become twisted, cutting off the blood supply and causing severe problems. This may be a result of a kick or blow to the testes or it can happen all on its own.

Symptoms Very similar to testicular trauma – agonising pain, sickness, dizziness, etc. However, the pain tends to be even more severe and only one testicle is involved. There is also usually obvious swelling and the pain and other symptoms come on rapidly and do not wear off after an hour. **This is a medical emergency and you should get to a doctor or a hospital A&E department as soon as possible.**

Treatment It is usually necessary to have a small operation to untwist the testicle and secure it with a stitch so it doesn't twist again. As long as this happens before the blood supply has been cut off for too long, there should be no long-term effects.

Problem Page

I've got these little white spots on my penis. Although I've never had sex I'm really scared it might be something terrible. I'm too embarrassed to tell anyone.

You can get spots on any part of your body – including your penis. In fact the warm, moist conditions around that area can be ideal for producing spots! If you have no pain or discharge (coloured leakage from your penis) it's unlikely to be anything to worry about. Make sure you wash every day, preferably with a mild, unscented soap and stick to cotton boxers rather than tight nylon underpants. And don't squeeze the spots! They should disappear within a few weeks.

My foreskin has always been a bit tight, but lately it seems to have got worse. It's red and swollen and although I can move it up and down a bit it won't go all the way back. What should I do?

This is a common problem in teenage boys. Your foreskin may not be loose enough to cope with your new large-size penis! Try easing it back gently using soap and water or baby oil. Sometimes this is enough to stretch the foreskin, but you should never force it or hurt yourself. Try gently every day for a couple of weeks. If it's not better by then, see your doctor.

Sometimes the foreskin becomes so tight that it constricts the blood flow to the end of the penis. The head then becomes red, swollen and extremely painful. **This is a medical emergency and you should either see a doctor or visit a hospital A&E department immediately.**

When I get a hard-on or if I'm masturbating I often notice a few drops of liquid dribbling out of the end of my penis. This often happens even if I don't ejaculate. I'm worried that it could mean I have a sexually transmitted infection.

It's normal for a healthy penis to produce a few drops of pre-ejaculatory fluid on erection and before ejaculation. This is usually clear or slightly milky and doesn't smell of anything much. As long as there's no blood or pus in the liquid and you aren't suffering from any itching or burning in your penis, there's no need to worry.

125

When I'm masturbating, just before I get to orgasm I feel my balls go all tight and hard. Why is this?

This is a normal part of ejaculation. Your testicles tighten and are pulled in and up towards your body. This helps force out the sperm and semen.

I have a pain in my right testicle. I've looked at them and they feel the same as always with no lumps or anything, but the pain has been there for three weeks. I do a lot of cycling – could that have anything to do with it?

Try taking a rest from cycling for a few days. If you feel better then you can assume that cycling is the problem. Try changing to a different type of saddle which puts less pressure on your testes. If the pain doesn't get any better make an appointment to check it with your GP.

Chapter 7

What Happens to Girls?

This chapter covers:

◇ How a girl's body changes during puberty
◇ Female sex organs
◇ Periods
◇ Hormones and emotions

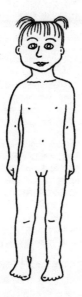

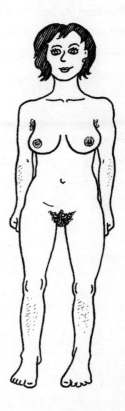

A girl's body changes from something like this . . .

. . . to something more like this

Girls go through puberty too – but you've probably noticed that already! Because some of the changes that happen – like developing breasts – are more obvious to the outside world, people often think that girls start puberty much earlier than boys. The truth is that they are on average only about a couple of months ahead.

Half of all girls will have noticed the first changes, such as a few pubic hairs or budding breasts, by the time they're 10, but it could be as early as 8 or as late as 14 or 15.

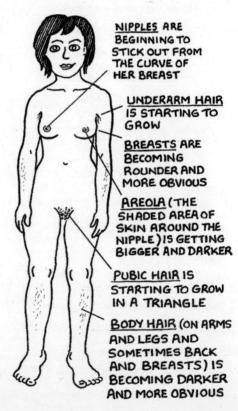

NIPPLES ARE BEGINNING TO STICK OUT FROM THE CURVE OF HER BREAST

UNDERARM HAIR IS STARTING TO GROW

BREASTS ARE BECOMING ROUNDER AND MORE OBVIOUS

AREOLA (THE SHADED AREA OF SKIN AROUND THE NIPPLE) IS GETTING BIGGER AND DARKER

PUBIC HAIR IS STARTING TO GROW IN A TRIANGLE

BODY HAIR (ON ARMS AND LEGS AND SOMETIMES BACK AND BREASTS) IS BECOMING DARKER AND MORE OBVIOUS

This is a picture of a girl who is about halfway through the changes of puberty

Growth Spurt

One of the most obvious changes for boys and girls is the growth spurt. In girls this starts at the beginning of puberty and it's often their feet which begin to get bigger first. Boys have their main growth spurt nearer the middle or end of puberty.

Breasts

Breasts are made up of a layer of fat covering a special sort of spongy tissue which has glands in it. These glands can eventually produce milk to feed a baby. Breast development starts with breast buds. These are tender, grape-sized lumps which grow behind each nipple. (Boys sometimes get these too!) Next, the area around the nipple (the *areola*) becomes darker. The breasts slowly get bigger and change shape to become more rounded. The whole process takes several years. During this time, most girls notice that their hips get bigger and their waist becomes more obvious. This makes them look more 'curvy'.

Pubic and Body Hair

Just like boys, girls start to grow hair under their arms, on their legs and around their sex organs. The first pubic hair is usually fine and soft, but it gradually spreads in a triangular shape over the area between the top of their legs, getting darker and curlier. Eventually the pubic hair can spread back towards the anus and onto the top part of the thighs.

Outer Sexual Organs

If you could see between a girl's legs it would look something like this:

OUTER LIPS (MEDICAL/LATIN NAME – LABIA MAJORIS) WHICH PROTECT THE SENSITIVE BITS INSIDE

INNER LIPS (MEDICAL/LATIN NAME – LABIA MINORA)

ANUS (OR BACK PASSAGE), WHERE STOOLS (SOLID WASTE OR POO) COME OUT

PUBIC HAIR, WHICH MAY STRETCH DOWN BETWEEN THE LEGS AND BACK TOWARDS THE ANUS

CLITORIS – THE TIP OF THE CLITORIS IS A SMALL, VERY SENSITIVE, FLESHY BUMP

URETHRA, WHERE URINE OR PEE COMES OUT

ENTRANCE TO THE VAGINA – THE TUBE THROUGH WHICH BLOOD FROM A PERIOD FLOWS AND THROUGH WHICH BABIES ARE BORN

She has three openings between her legs, the urethra, vagina and anus – although the opening of the urethra is so small it can be difficult to see. Stools are passed through the anus and urine comes out of the urethra. The *vagina* is the opening where blood from a period flows out and is also the sex passage where the penis is inserted during sex, as well as the birth canal through which babies are born.

Changes on the Inside

Important changes take place inside a girl's body where they can't be seen. These are the changes to the reproductive organs – the parts of the body which produce eggs and allow a baby to form and develop. This diagram shows you where the different reproductive organs are:

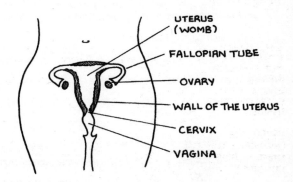

Girls have two ovaries, each containing thousands of tiny eggs. After puberty, one or two of these eggs are released each month. The ovaries are also important because they produce the hormones which control the cycle of a girl's periods. Boys and girls share some of the same hormones, but there are also special and very different male and female hormones. For boys the most important one is testosterone and for girls there are two – *oestrogen* and *progesterone*. But, for both sexes, hormones that make you grow and change can also affect your emotions.

Periods

Most girls start to have periods at about 13 – but they can start as early as 8 or as late as 18. They might not happen very often at first, but, after a year or so, most girls have a period about once a month. Women carry on having them until they're around 50.

The female hormones, oestrogen and progesterone, control the release of eggs by the ovaries. At around 12 to 14 most girls start to release an egg each month. It travels along the fallopian tube towards the uterus. If it meets a sperm along the way, it might be fertilised. A fertilised egg can grow more cells and can nestle into the wall of the uterus and develop into a tiny foetus. The lining of the uterus gets thicker each month so it can support and nourish a growing foetus if necessary. If the foetus carries on growing, it eventually becomes a baby. But usually the egg is not fertilised before it gets to the uterus. Then it starts to break up and, at the same time, the lining of the uterus begins to break away into little pieces. This mixture of blood, dead cells and the remains of the egg slowly flows out of the girl's vagina. This is what makes a period.

As soon as one period is over, the hormone levels start to build up again making the lining of the uterus get thicker. Soon another egg is released and the whole cycle is repeated.

Girls use towels or tampons to soak up the blood. You have probably

Sanitary towels or pads

seen them in the chemists or in your own
bathroom at home.

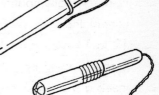

Girls can also have problems
with their periods. They may
get tummy aches, back ache
and feel really tired and miserable.

Hormones and Emotions

Tampons

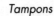

There are three important initials
here – PMS!

They stand for 'Pre-Menstrual Syndrome'. Many girls
and women get very fed-up and miserable for 3 or
4 days before a period starts. This is caused by the
hormones whizzing about. They may tend to cry about
'nothing' or seem unreasonable or angry or just unpredictable. They often feel awful with tummy ache, a
bloated feeling and sometimes tender breasts too. They

A Good Tip

If your girlfriend or one of your girl friends is having
a period, she may not feel like going swimming or
doing anything very sporty. And she could be too
shy to tell you why she doesn't feel 100% fit. She
will be really impressed if you guess what the
problem is without her having to spell it out – and
without you telling everyone else!

---

may get more spots (acne) at this time of the month. They need lots of sympathy and understanding.

Problem Page

What does it feel like for girls having breasts? Do they hurt?

Most girls don't have any particular problems with their breasts, but when they first appear, it can take some getting used to. They may feel tender and swollen around the time she has her period and running or playing sport can be uncomfortable if it makes them jiggle around! Wearing a well-fitted bra or a special sports bra gives them more support.

How much blood does a girl lose during her period? Isn't it bad for her?

A girl or woman usually loses between a tablespoonful and a small teacupful of blood in one period, that is, once a month. However, it can often seem a lot more than this because the blood is mixed with old cells from the broken-up lining of her uterus plus some mucus from her cervix.

Her body can usually replace the amount of blood lost well before her next period, but, because red blood cells are so important to health, she needs to ensure she eats a good varied diet that contains plenty of iron. Some girls suffer from very frequent and/or very heavy periods and the loss of red blood cells can make them anaemic. They might feel tired, faint and look very pale. A girl suffering

134

from anaemia would probably need help from her doctor to boost the iron in her blood and regulate her periods.

Do girls think about sex as much as boys?

There's no easy answer to that but teenage girls certainly do think about sex – a lot! Just as boys are affected by their hormones, so girls become more aware of all the references to sex that are going on around them and their own bodies' response to it. They are often very curious about sex, but it's possible they think about it in a different way from boys. Female biology and our society make it very clear to a girl that she is the one at risk of pregnancy. It's partly for this reason that many girls think about sex more in terms of relationships and romance than simple physical pleasure.

Do girls masturbate?

Many do – but it's probably not as common as it is with boys. Boys grow up touching their penis every day – when they get dressed or go to the loo – so they quickly realise that holding or touching it in a certain way feels very good. Many girls are more nervous about their own bodies and feel that it's somehow wrong to touch themselves 'down there'. However once they do, they're able to give themselves sexual pleasure through masturbation in much the same way that a boy can.

Chapter 8

Sex

This chapter covers:
- ◇ The mechanics of sex
- ◇ The dangers of getting 'carried away'
- ◇ Sex – the first time
- ◇ Sex and the law
- ◇ When is it normal to start having sex?
- ◇ Contraception and condom use
- ◇ Unwanted pregnancy
- ◇ Sexually transmitted infections (STIs)
- ◇ Other types of sexuality
- ◇ Sex abuse and male rape
- ◇ Common problems with sex

If you've read the earlier chapters of this book, you'll already know a bit about how boys' and girls' sexual parts work. However, if you've just turned to this chapter you might need to refer back either now or later to help you understand some of the basic biology.

The Mechanics of Sex

When a man and a woman become sexually excited, the man's penis grows hard and erect and the woman's vagina starts to produce a natural, slippery lubrication. When the man puts his penis into her vagina he feels the muscles in the walls of the vagina grip around him. This feels very warm and exciting. By moving their bodies together, and the man thrusting his penis in and out, he will (often very quickly) reach an orgasm and ejaculate. The sperm will shoot up into the woman's vagina and start their journey through her uterus and into the fallopian tubes in search of an egg to fertilise.

This is called *sexual intercourse*. At its simplest, it's nothing more than a penis going inside a vagina and can be over in as little as 10 seconds. *Making love* is something else. This is based on a relationship with caring, trust and joint responsibility.

More Than Intercourse

In a caring and equal relationship a couple would talk about sex before it happened, discuss any fears or worries they have and make sure they take precautions to prevent unwanted pregnancy or the spread of sexually transmitted infections (STIs). They would also take time to get to know each other well first. This includes becoming familiar with each other's bodies. All the kissing and hugging, petting, stroking and feeling that can go on in the early stage of a relationship is excellent practice for making love – but it also feels very good in its own right!

DOC BOX
Female Orgasm

Sexual intercourse doesn't necessarily involve orgasm for the woman. She may have one, but in biological terms, intercourse is just as successful (is just as likely to make her pregnant) whether she does or not.

This is often a disappointment to young people, particularly if the boy reaches his orgasm very fast. Learning how to touch her, either before or after intercourse, especially around the clitoris where she is most sensitive, helps give her pleasure as well.

The Dangers of Getting 'Carried Away'

Unfortunately, people sometimes forget to talk about sex and precautions with their partner. Many young people write to problem pages or appear at clinics explaining, 'One thing led to another and we just got carried away'. The obvious dangers are unwanted pregnancies and infections, but there's an emotional danger too. Because sex does feel so good and so exciting, it is easy – for boys *and* girls – in the heat of the moment to go further than they meant to. When you're on the point of having sex, there's nothing more important or attractive than the person you are with. But afterwards it can be a shock to discover you don't know them very well – and may not even like them very much!

Most surveys suggest that girls and boys start to think about sex at around the same age. However, this may not seem very obvious. Girls are often more cautious than boys because they are well aware that it is *they* who run the risk of an unwanted pregnancy, not the boy. Plus there is a common double standard towards sex: a boy who sleeps with a girl and then moves on to another partner right afterwards is seen as a stud or a bit of a lad. He may even boast about it. A girl in the same situation gets a reputation for being easy or even a bit of a slag or tart. One is supposed to be good and the other bad – yet they've both done the same thing.

Another problem is that boys and girls (and men and women) often have different emotional reactions to sex. To some boys, particularly if they're immature, sex is all that matters and the girl is only a means to an end. Something to boast about. But to many girls, having sex means a real emotional commitment and they assume it's the same for the boy. If he acts coldly or goes off her afterwards, she's very hurt and confused, and feels betrayed. Boys who do this a lot quickly gain the reputation of *users* amongst girls. And, because girls talk to each other about this sort of thing more than boys, word spreads so that other girls learn to steer clear and distrust them.

The First Time

Everyone's first time is different and, for some, it can be very disappointing. Making sure that both of you are ready for this step (and that means *talking* about it), getting contraception and protection sorted out (*talking* again) and ensuring you have somewhere safe, private and comfortable will all help. Understanding the following can also make a difference:

◇ Most boys get over-excited the first time and ejaculate too quickly. Waiting and trying again (or masturbating alone beforehand) can help.

◇ Girls very often take longer than boys to become sexually aroused. Foreplay (kissing, stroking, touching) helps.

◇ The first time can be painful for girls and they may bleed – a lot. This can be scary and upsetting for both of you. Try taking things slowly and give her lots of reassurance.

Sex and the Law

The age of consent for male–female (heterosexual) sex is 16 in England, Scotland and Wales and 17 in Northern Ireland. This is the age at which the law says a girl is able to make a fully informed and properly thought-out decision about whether she's willing to have sex.

It is an offence for any male to have sex with a girl under the age of consent. If the pair have been going out for a while, she is nearly 16 and he is not much older, then, as long as she genuinely did agree to sex, the chances of prosecution are very low. However, some angry parents do make a fuss and the police can be involved, which is difficult and upsetting for everyone.

If the boy is older than 17 and the girl is not yet 16, then the situation is much more serious. He could be prosecuted and get up to two years in prison. If the girl he has sex with is under 13, then technically he could receive life

DOC BOX
Age of Consent for Getting Advice on Sex

Even if you and/or your girlfriend are under 16, doctors still have to keep anything you tell them private – just as they would for an adult. (The only exception to this would be if one of you was in danger of serious harm or abuse.) This means you can get help from a doctor or a young people's clinic, like a Brook or a Family Planning clinic without the consent or knowledge of your parents or carers.

Doctors and clinics can also provide free contraception when necessary.

imprisonment (25 years). If the boy is under 17 he can't be prosecuted, but could be placed in care.

The age of consent for male–male (homosexual) sex is also 16 in England, Scotland and Wales.

When Is It Normal to Start Having Sex?

This is very difficult to say. Many surveys have been carried out, but people don't always tell the truth! However, it seems that the average age for having intercourse for the first time is about 17, but it's gradually getting younger.

One recent survey, which only asked people under 20 when they'd first had sex, suggested that 60% of them had done it by the time they were 16. But another piece of research looking at young male university students suggested that at least one third of them were still virgins.

Who's Telling the Truth?

Studies that ask young people when they had sex *and* when they thought their friends started doing it always seem to show that 'the friends' start earlier. This suggests that there's a lot of boasting or wishful thinking going on! Unfortunately it puts pressure on young people by making them think that everyone else is doing it – so they need to start too.

Research does show that the younger you are when you start having sex:

◇ the less likely you are to use precautions against pregnancy and infection
◇ the more likely you are to regret it or feel bad afterwards

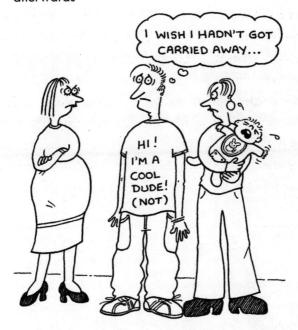

Contraception

Contraception or birth control means anything which prevents or reduces the risk of pregnancy. There are many different sorts of contraception but only one, the condom, is designed for use by the man. So, when it comes to you taking responsibility for birth control, you might not have

Tips on Using Condoms

No form of contraception is 100% reliable, but problems are often due to user-error. This is particularly true for condoms so, for maximum safety, follow these tips:

◇ Stick to well-known, reliable brands – novelty condoms in funny shapes and colours might be amusing, but they don't necessarily work very well.
◇ Don't keep them where they can be punctured, for example in your pocket with keys.
◇ Open the foil pack carefully – don't risk tearing the condom with teeth or nails.
◇ Sounds obvious, but make sure you've put it on the right way up!

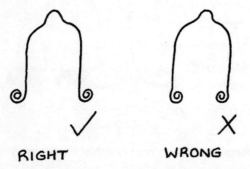

RIGHT   WRONG

◇ Pinch the little teat at the end of the condom before putting it on. This squeezes the air out, leaving space for your semen.

◇ Put the condom on the head of your penis and roll it down gently until the whole penis is covered.

◇ Put it on as soon as your penis is erect, *before* you start to have sex. There are often a few drops of semen on the end of your penis before ejaculation and if this gets into your girlfriend's vagina she could get pregnant.

◇ After you've reached ejaculation you need to pull your penis out while it is still erect. Hold the condom tight against the base of your penis while you do this – so there's no risk of it spilling inside her body.

◇ Remove the condom, tie a knot in the end and throw it away wrapped in a tissue or something. Don't try to flush it down the loo – they float!

◇ Always carry a spare in case you damage the first one – or want to make love again!

IMPORTANT – using baby oil or hand creams can feel great during masturbation but **never** use them with a condom. Oil-based products attack the latex in condoms causing them to tear and break – often leading to unwanted pregnancies.

much choice, but condoms do have very definite advantages. They're:

◇ safe
◇ reliable
◇ available

Because they are a simple barrier method, which prevents sperm from reaching an egg, they don't involve drugs or medication. So (with the rare exception of allergic reactions to the spermicide on some condoms) they don't carry the risk of side effects. When used properly they are very reliable, and they're easily available from shops, machines in public lavatories and free from Family Planning and young people's health clinics.

But their biggest advantage is they not only act as birth control, they also give protection against sexually transmitted infections (STIs). By using a condom you're showing that you care. You're taking responsibility and protecting both you and your partner.

Even if your girlfriend is on the Pill, you should still use a condom. This is sometimes called the *Double Dutch* method. It may seem like overkill but it cuts down the risk of pregnancy, proves that you're man enough to share responsibility, and protects both of you from infection.

For more information about other forms of contraception and advice on where to get it, look in the Contacts section at the end of this book.

Emergency Contraception

Emergency contraception (sometimes called the 'Morning After Pill') can be used up to 72 hours (3 days) after unprotected sex. It consists of artificial hormones in the form of pills, which a girl can take to stop an egg that may have been fertilised from growing into a baby.

If you do get carried away and have unprotected sex or if something goes wrong with your contraception, for example, your condom splits or tears, then emergency contraception can be very useful. **But it does not prevent sexually transmitted infections (STIs).**

Emergency contraception is available free from family doctors, Family Planning clinics and special young people's clinics. Or, if the girl is over 16, she can buy it from a pharmacist. Although it's effective, it is not 100% reliable, particularly if she does not take it until the second or third day after sex. It should **never** be used as a regular method of contraception.

Unwanted Pregnancy

The UK has the highest rate of unwanted and unplanned teenage pregnancy in Europe. There are many possible reasons for this, but often, the boy and girl concerned have assumed that it just can't happen to them. But it *can* and it *does*!

A girl is at her most fertile when she ovulates (releases an egg). This usually happens roughly halfway between her periods, but it can vary a lot, particularly in younger girls – so you can't rely on any time in the month being

Myths About Pregnancy

She can't get pregnant if we do it standing up.

YES SHE CAN

She can't get pregnant the first time we have sex.

YES SHE CAN

She can't get pregnant if she goes to the loo or washes out her vagina afterwards.

YES SHE CAN

She can't get pregnant if she doesn't have an orgasm.

YES SHE CAN

She can't get pregnant if I take my penis out before I ejaculate or I don't put my penis all the way in.

YES SHE CAN

She can't get pregnant if we have sex during her period.

IT'S UNLIKELY, BUT NOT IMPOSSIBLE

Believing in any of these can seriously alter your life. If you don't want a child, don't trust to luck. Either don't have sex or make sure you use a reliable method of contraception.

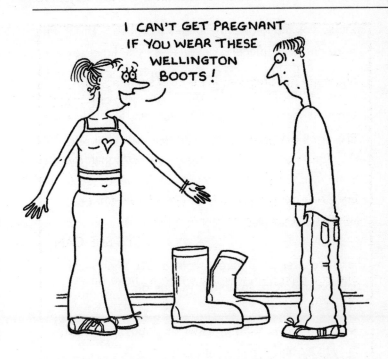

'safe'. If your girlfriend thinks she might be pregnant (the first sign is usually a missed period) she needs to talk to a doctor straight away. You can support her in this by helping her make an appointment with her family doctor or a special young people's clinic like a Brook or Family Planning clinic. There are also special helplines for young people in this situation (see the Contacts section).

Sexually Transmitted Infections

Sexually transmitted infections (STIs) are passed on either through intercourse or just through touching each other's sexual parts. Most can be cleared up easily with antibiotics, but sometimes the symptoms are mild or hard to spot, so you may not know there's a problem. This means you're at risk of infecting anyone else you have sex with.

Some STIs, like gonorrhoea or syphilis, seemed to be on the decrease about 10 years ago, but they are now becoming much more common. Others, like chlamydia, were almost unheard of 10 years ago, but are now reaching near-epidemic proportions. Chlamydia often has no symptoms, but, if left untreated, can cause serious damage in women and is one of the major causes of infertility in later life.

There are over 25 different types of STI. Their most common symptoms in boys and men are:

◇ discharge – could be clear or cloudy, white or yellow and possibly smelly
◇ pain or burning sensation when you pee
◇ rash, itching, lumps, sores or blisters on or around the penis
◇ pain in the penis or testes – particularly during sex
◇ nothing! A boy may have an STI without any symptoms or signs yet be infectious and able to pass it on to his sexual partner(s)

If you think you may have an STI, even if you are symptom-free, you'll need to get help and advice – quickly! This usually means a trip to a special or GUM clinic. For further information see Chapter 9 and look at the Contacts section at the end of the book.

Better Safe Than Sorry

If you're thinking about having sex with someone, remember — there's no way to tell whether or not they have an STI. Perhaps they don't know themselves, or maybe they do know but don't want to admit it.

The only ways to protect yourself are:

◇ not to have sex
◇ to avoid penetration (intercourse) or any direct genital contact which could transfer body fluids,. concentrating on touching, stroking and rubbing 'safe' body areas instead
◇ to use a condom or another barrier method of contraception, such as the female condom (Femidom)

Anything else and you're putting yourself – and possibly your partner – at risk.

HIV

HIV (the virus that causes AIDS) doesn't cause any symptoms at all. Although it's often associated with gay sex, more and more people are now being infected through heterosexual (male–female) sex. If you think you're at risk, the only way to know for sure is to have an HIV test, but it can take three to six months after infection before a test is accurate.

Other Risk Factors

Making clear and sensible decisions about sex can be hard enough when you're thinking straight. Adding alcohol or drugs to the equation means you're more likely to make mistakes and take dangerous risks. Many young people have their first experience of sex while they or their partner are drunk. They are less likely to use any precautions and more likely to regret it afterwards. Taking drugs can also affect your judgement so you do things or make decisions that are dangerous or risky.

Alcohol and drugs have another effect too. Drinking too much or using Class A drugs like heroin and amphetamines can stop you getting an erection. You may feel like having sex, but your penis won't do what you want it to do.

Other Types of Sexuality

Although this chapter mainly deals with male–female sex, not all boys are attracted to girls and for some young men, sex isn't much of an issue at all. Some boys know from an early age that they are gay or homosexual and are only ever attracted to other boys. Some people are bisexual, having feelings for and relationships with partners of both sexes before perhaps settling into a longer-term relationship. And some enjoy close friendships but don't have any sexual desires. These are all normal, but *any* kind of active sexual relationship will carry some

152

risk. A boy may not be able to make his male partner pregnant, but there is a higher risk of sexually transmitted infection in gay sex. It's just as important to use a condom. For more information about homosexuality see Chapter 4 and the Contacts section.

Abuse and Male Rape

Many people assume that sexual abuse or rape is something that only happens to girls or women, but boys and men are also at risk of unwanted and sometimes violent sexual attacks. Sex abusers target children and young people of either sex and in very many cases are family members or friends. They may spend a long time getting to know their victims and 'persuading' them (often with threats or bribes) to cooperate. Male rape can involve an attack or violence from a stranger or strangers, or from someone the victim knows. In either case, victims often feel ashamed of or responsible for what has happened and this can prevent them reporting the crime and/or asking for help. Rapists and abusers rely on this fear factor. If you have been abused or sexually attacked it's very important you tell someone you trust. This might be your school nurse, teacher or GP, or you can contact a young people's clinic or a special helpline like ChildLine, the NSPCC or Survivors UK (see the Contacts section for more information).

Common Problems With Sex

There's no way you could talk to your friends about problems with sex – but it was always a relief to find that

153

other people suffered as well. For example, when I first started seeing girls I sometimes got premature ejaculation – or couldn't do it at all. I'd feel all fuelled up but nothing was happening. This went on for about two years and I thought that was it for life. I was all bravado – but shit-scared inside. A couple of relationships ended because the girls wanted to have sex and I really led them on even though I knew I couldn't follow through.

Geoff, 25

Premature ejaculation

This is something that happens to all boys and men at some time! It basically means coming too quickly or reaching an orgasm before you want to. It's usually caused by a combination of anxiety and over-enthusiasm.

Symptoms Particularly common when you first start to have sex or have sex with a new partner, you find that you ejaculate almost immediately when you start lovemaking.

Treatment Understanding that it's normal can be enough to help you relax and get over it. But unfortunately, the more you worry the more likely it is to happen. Practising masturbation while concentrating on the feelings that you get just before orgasm can help you recognise them and delay them – either by stopping the sexual stimulation for a short while or by thinking about something that has absolutely nothing to do with sex, such as trying to remember your mum's birthday or counting backwards from 100 in threes. For more information on places where you can get more help and advice see the Contacts section.

Failure to get an erection

This is rarely a problem for young men, so when it does happen, it can be a shock.

Symptoms If you never get an erection, even on masturbation or first waking in the morning, then you should see your doctor as this could be a symptom of a serious problem.

If you normally have erections but your penis fails you when you're about to have sex, it's probably due to nerves.

Treatment Taking things slowly and spending more time kissing, touching, stroking and hugging your partner (sometimes called foreplay) before intercourse can help. For information on where to get further advice see the Contacts section at the end of the book.

Pain in the penis during sex

This could be a symptom of several problems, but in young men, it's most likely the result of over-use.

Symptoms Discomfort or stinging or swelling and redness during or after masturbation or sexual intercourse.

Treatment If you think you might have been overdoing it, give your penis a rest for a few days. Using lubrication like KY Jelly or saliva can help.

If there is redness or swelling of the foreskin you may be suffering from para-phimosis (see Chapter 6).

Pain in the testes when you can't have sex

Sometimes called blue balls, this is caused by the increased blood flow to the testes during sexual arousal.

Symptoms When you become sexually excited, your testicles can increase in size by 25% to 50%, often turning a bluish colour. This makes them ache or feel uncomfortable.

After orgasm and ejaculation, the testes (like the penis) quickly return to their normal size, but if you don't have sex this takes longer to happen and the discomfort can last for about half an hour. However, it is not dangerous or harmful and should not be used as a form of emotional blackmail to persuade your partner to have sex!

Treatment None necessary!

Problem Page

Will my penis be big enough to satisfy a girl?

Boys and men are far more worried than girls about penis size! The most sensitive areas of a girl's sexual parts are the lower third of her vagina and the area outside it, particularly around and on the clitoris. There are fewer nerve endings around the top of the vagina so having a really long penis doesn't make much difference. It really is a matter of what you do with it that counts!

What position is best for sex?

There are many different possible (and some seemingly impossible) positions, but, particularly for beginners, the best ones are the easiest and the most comfortable. The boy lying on top of the girl with his legs between hers allows him to take his weight on his forearms so she doesn't get squashed. It also lets them look at each other and kiss. She can open her legs wider and pull her knees up or tilt her bottom to alter the angle of penetration so it feels as good as possible for her.

I want to use a condom but I'm scared it will make my erection disappear if I put one on.

This is a common fear with an easy answer. Practise first! Buy yourself a pack of condoms and try putting them on. You'll soon get used to the feel of them and you'll be much more confident in opening the pack and putting one on when you are about to make love. Remember – it's important to put the condom on before there's any kind of sexual contact.

Surely it's safe to have sex as long as I pull my penis out before I come?

Pulling your penis out before you come or ejaculate is known as the 'withdrawal method'. It doesn't work! Apart from being very difficult to do reliably, your penis usually leaks a drop or two of semen when it's erect but before you ejaculate. Even these tiny drops can contain millions of sperm – more than enough to get a girl pregnant. Many couples have been caught out this way.

How can a girl tell she's pregnant?

The most usual signs of pregnancy are a missed period

followed by feelings of sickness and sore breasts. But not everyone gets these and some girls continue having periods through at least part of their pregnancy. Also, the fear of being pregnant can be enough to make a girl feel queasy – or even delay her period. So there's no reliable way to tell from symptoms alone. If a girl thinks there's a risk she could be pregnant, i.e., if she's had unprotected sex, then she needs to have a pregnancy test as soon as possible. You can buy DIY pregnancy test kits from supermarkets and chemists, but it's much better to go to a doctor or clinic where they can do the test and give advice and help. There's more information on this in Chapter 9.

Do girls have erections?

Some people might think this is a silly question, but the answer is yes – they do! When boys get excited extra blood flows to their sexual organs, filling up the penis and making it hard. The same thing happens with girls. As they become aroused, the blood fills up and darkens their labia (the lips around the vagina) and makes the clitoris harder and more sensitive.

Why do we have orgasms?

Orgasms have two main purposes. First of all they feel really good, so they make people want to have sex. In biological terms this helps the species reproduce – although that might not be the main thing on *your* mind!

158

Orgasm is the effect of a series of muscular spasms. In men this pushes the sperm and semen out of the body through the penis and into the woman. A woman's vagina and uterus also have a series of contractions during orgasm and this can help the sperm travel up to find an egg. But, because the sperm are capable of doing this on their own anyway, she could still get pregnant whether or not she has an orgasm.

If I have sex with my girlfriend will she be able to tell that I'm still a virgin?

Does it matter? Perhaps you've boasted a bit so she thinks you're much more experienced than you really are. If so, this is as likely to scare her as reassure her. But she probably won't know the truth unless you tell her. First time sex with any partner can be awkward and embarrassing, and the best way of coping is to talk and laugh about it together. If you want her to think you really know what you're doing, take it slowly, make sure you're both ready and sort out contraception and protection beforehand. That will really impress her!

Chapter 9

Getting Help

This chapter covers:
- ◇ Why you might choose to get further help
- ◇ Choosing someone to talk to
- ◇ Telephone helplines
- ◇ Doctors and other health professionals
- ◇ Your rights to confidentiality
- ◇ Young people's health and advice clinics
- ◇ Special clinics

Although all the changes which happen during puberty are a normal part of growing up, most people find they need a bit of help and advice at some time. Perhaps you just want to ask your dad about the best sort of razor to buy, or check out with your older brother or best friend which anti-spot lotions they recommend. Often you might already know the answers to these questions, but talking it through with someone else and knowing that they agree can make you feel a lot more confident. However, there may come a time when you have a more serious or personal problem which you don't want to ask your parents or your best friend about. This is when you need to think about talking to an adult outside the family, maybe a teacher or a doctor, or using an advice line.

Sometimes it's possible to tell if friends are going through, or thinking, the same things. Then it becomes quite easy to talk to them and a real relief. But if it was anything serious I'd prefer talking to a school counsellor, perhaps from fear of rejection from my friends or of feeling insecure.   Tony, 21

There's no way you talk to friends about anything personal or body stuff. It's just not something you could or would want to talk about. Girls do but guys don't.
                                                                                                    James, 16

Boys talk about football, booze and girls. We can't express feelings to each other because we'd look like 'sissies'. Now I've got a girlfriend who I can chat to about problems.   Mark, 15

No one finds it easy to talk about the things that worry them most. But finding out that someone can listen, is prepared to take you seriously and does want to help really will make a difference. Research suggests that boys do find it harder to talk about emotions than girls, so they might not always get the support they need from those around them. Sometimes this leads to serious problems like depression and there's a worryingly high rate of suicide among boys and young men.

Young Men and Suicide

◇ 26% of all deaths of young men aged 20 to 24 in the UK are a result of suicide.

◇ This compares with only 1% of all deaths in the general population.

◇ Over 700 young people aged between 15 and 24 die by suicide every year in the UK.

◇ 4 out of 5 of them are young men.

Talking to Friends

While you might not want to broadcast your innermost problems, talking a worry through with a good and trusted friend can definitely help. Putting your feelings into words helps you work out your priorities and put things into perspective. The advantages of friends are that you already know them, they're usually around when you need them and they've often had similar experiences to yours. They'll almost certainly be sympathetic (and sometimes that's all you need), but they might not have all the answers you're looking for.

Talking to Adults

Adults don't necessarily have all the answers either, but they do usually have more experience. If you choose your person carefully, you should get the sort of help or reassurance you need. Obvious people include your parents or your favourite teacher, but you should also consider your best friend's mum or dad, a school nurse, family doctor, youth club leader, sports coach or pharmacist.

Choosing Someone to Talk to

Obviously you're not going to talk to someone unless you feel you can trust them – but you also need to warn them you're asking for serious help in case they feel uncomfortable with the situation.

Make this clear by asking if you can talk to them about something important and personal. This gives them a chance to find some quiet time and space where the two of you can chat in private.

Ask whether they're prepared to keep whatever you say confidential (private) to the two of you. This might be very important to you but it's often a difficult thing for a grown-up to agree to. They might want to know more about the problem first or, particularly in the case of a teacher or another person who works professionally with young people, they might need to warn you that there are some things they *can't* promise to keep secret. For example, if you were in danger of being abused or injured, they would have to pass this information on to Social Services.

Talking to Telephone Helplines

Telephone helplines or advice lines can be a very good first point of contact for medium to serious problems. Most of them guarantee confidentiality, but, whether they do or not, it's up to you how much you tell them. And if you chose not to give them your name or address they wouldn't be able to pass that information on, even if they wanted to. People call them with all sorts of problems. It could be anything from advice on making up with your best mate after a row, to support while your mum and dad's marriage falls apart; or confidential information and advice on a problem you're having with your willy, to crisis support if you (or your best mate) felt depressed and suicidal.

Choosing a Helpline

Although most helplines are genuine and professionally run, a few of them act as fronts for commercial, religious or political organisations that are more interested in getting your money or changing your point of view than helping you with your problem.

When choosing a helpline follow these tips:

◇ Pick a well-known national or local helpline – or one that has been personally recommended to you by someone (see the Contacts section at the back of the book for our suggestions).

Most helplines go for the 'listening ear' approach. This means they encourage the caller to talk about whatever it is that worries them. They might ask some direct questions or just make sympathetic noises, but their experience tells them that the priority for many callers is to talk about their problem knowing that someone is listening to and accepting their story. Helpline counsellors always have some training and, with the major helplines like ChildLine, the Samaritans or Brook, they also have on-going supervision. Their counsellors understand how difficult it is to make that first call and know that many young people will probably ring several times before they can talk about what it is that's really worrying them.

◇ If in doubt check they are a member of the Telephone Helplines Association (THA) – this means they guarantee to offer non-judgemental advice.

◇ Avoid any helpline which charges a 'premium' telephone rate – they're going to be more interested in getting your money than in helping you with your problem.

◇ If the person at the other end sounds more interested in getting your personal details or making you feel bad about yourself, make your excuses and hang up.

Advantages and Disadvantages of Talking to Helplines

Advantages	Disadvantages
◇ You're in control – you can hang up any time you want. ◇ You don't need to give your name or any other details if you don't choose to. ◇ Sometimes all you need is reassurance.	◇ You don't know the person you're talking to. ◇ Sometimes the lines can be very busy and you can't get through easily. ◇ Sometimes they can't give you direct help unless they know who and where you are and the full story.

But

Their biggest advantage is that they help you take a step towards getting one-to-one support and advice. Helplines can often suggest very practical ways of doing this. They have lists of local resources and they can also help you rehearse ways to talk to someone closer to home about your problem.

Some helplines will simply listen and help you sort out your own priorities or course of action. Others will make direct suggestions, while some can refer you to local sources of help or will be prepared to take action on your behalf – with your consent. For more information about who offers what, have a look in the Contacts section at the end of the book.

Talking to Doctors and Other Health Professionals

School nurses

If your school is lucky enough to have one (numbers vary across the UK) your school nurse is a brilliant person for practical face-to-face advice, particularly about problems to do with growing up or your body. For example, if you're worried that you aren't growing as fast as other people or you're bothered by lumps or aches, talking to your school nurse can often put your mind at rest. She'll either be able to reassure you or tell you that you do need to get some further help, perhaps from your family doctor. She can also give useful suggestions on coping with spots, skin care and diet, etc. Generally any discussion will be confidential unless you are in danger of being abused or injured. In this case she would have to tell the head teacher and Social Services. If your school does not have a school nurse, it might have a school counsellor. They will tend to deal with emotional problems rather than health worries, but they can point you in the right direction.

Pharmacists

A pharmacist is the person (often in a white coat) who is in charge of giving out the medicines in a chemist's shop. They may not seem like the obvious person to ask, but they've had professional training in how drugs and medicines work and can give you excellent advice on subjects like skin care, excess sweating, smelly feet, headaches and general aches and pains. Of course it's a bit nerve-wracking talking about your personal symptoms in front of lots of other people. What you can do is wait your turn in the queue then ask if you can speak to the pharmacist in private. Most pharmacies have a quiet area where you can talk and get advice without other customers overhearing. They can often answer any immediate worries and suggest the best type of over-the-counter medicine or pain relief if you need it. Or they may tell you that you need to see your doctor.

Doctors

Although most problems and worries can usually be solved, there are times when it's important to talk to a doctor. This may seem scary or embarrassing, but GPs (family doctors) are very used to dealing with all the worries and confusions which go with growing up. They'll be happy to help put your mind at rest. And they'd usually much prefer you asked them for advice – even about something very simple – than worry about it on your own.

Some GP practices have rules about how old you have to be before you can see a doctor on your own. If you're

DOC BOX
Always See a Doctor if You Have . . .

◇ a severe, prolonged pain in any part of the body
◇ a mole that changes shape, colour, size or bleeds
   or gets itchy – possible sign of early stage of skin
   cancer (malignant melanoma)
◇ blood in urine or semen
◇ smelly discharge from the penis
◇ a hard lump or swelling in the scrotum/testes
◇ sudden weight loss when you haven't been trying
   to lose weight – possible sign of serious disease
◇ severe headache and/or stiff neck, high
   temperature and a blotchy rash on your body or
   limbs which doesn't fade when you press a glass
   against it – this could be meningitis. **This is a
   medical emergency; see your doctor or get to a
   hospital A&E department as soon as possible.**

Of course you can also ask about all sorts of other
worries.

not sure about yours, you could ring the receptionist and
ask. Many doctors are very aware that young people will
want to talk about things in private and often try to make
it easy for them. For example, when you visit for something
like a sore throat or ear infection they might suggest your

mum waits outside for a few minutes. This gives you a chance to talk about anything that's been worrying you.

> ## One Doctor Told Us:
>
> At our practice we try to make sure that anyone over the age of about 12 has the chance to talk to a doctor or nurse if they want to. When they come in for something routine like a throat infection, we often suggest that they pop back a week later on their own just so we can check they're getting better. This gives us a chance to ask if there's anything else worrying them and helps the young person to get used to talking to us without feeling everything has to be said through their mum or dad.

Changing Your Doctor

Once you're 16 you can choose your own doctor. You might prefer to see a different doctor in the same surgery or move to a new practice altogether.

◇ If you want to change to a different doctor in the same surgery, just ask the receptionist.
◇ If you want to change to a new practice, just call in at that practice and they will give you the forms to fill in. You don't have to tell your old doctor why you want to move.

Doctors and Your Right to Confidentiality

Although you can't usually change or choose your own doctor until you are 16, even if you're under this age everything you tell your doctor should be kept confidential. This means that they won't repeat it to your parents or anyone else without your permission.

The only exception to this is if you are in danger of being injured or abused. In this case the doctor has a legal duty to inform Social Services that you are at risk, but most doctors will warn you of this ahead of time and discuss the procedure with you.

Confidentiality also applies to talking about sex. Although it is illegal for a boy or man to have sex with a girl who is under 16, your doctor should still be able to advise you and offer you or your girlfriend free birth control.

If you are in any doubt, ask your doctor before you start if your talk will be confidential or private. They should be able to reassure you.

Young People's Health and Advice Clinics

In some areas, particularly in large towns, there are special clinics for young people (usually up to the age of 25) that offer free, confidential help for problems. Sometimes these are purely counselling clinics, but many also offer medical or contraceptive help. You can usually find them in the local phone book under *Clinics* or *Counselling* or look in the Contacts section in this book for central telephone numbers that can give you details of local services.

The advantage of attending a special young people's clinic is that you're unlikely to run into your mum or next-door neighbour in the waiting room and all the staff there are experienced in dealing with younger clients. You'll be treated as an adult but the clinic will probably feel a lot more friendly and relaxed than your GP's surgery. Many clinics also offer a drop-in service where you don't have to make an appointment.

Special Clinics or GUMs

GUM stands for *genito-urinary medicine*. These are some-times called *special clinics*, they're usually attached to large hospitals and they offer free and confidential help for sexually transmitted infections (STIs). To find your nearest one, ring Sexwise (see Contacts section) and then contact the clinic to find out whether you need to make an appointment or if they offer a drop-in service. Although it's obviously embarrassing and scary to think that you might have an STI, these clinics are very matter-of-fact and reassuring and will give you advice plus any medication you need. They are also able to offer appointments to anyone else you have had sex with, as they usually need to be treated as well.

And Finally . . .

Although this book talks a lot about the problems you can have with growing up, it's important to remember that most people cope very well without any major difficulties. We hope that you will have found the answers to most of your questions in our book, but if there is still something worrying you, there is always somewhere to get help. If you don't feel able to talk to your parents, doctor or any of the other grown-ups we've suggested – or if they can't answer your questions – do try one of the organisations, helplines or websites listed in the Contacts section.

Contacts

The following organisations, websites and helplines can give you free and confidential advice and information.

Note – *numbers beginning '080' or '0500' are Freephone and don't show up on phone bills.*

For medical queries and advice on whether or not a symptom is a medical emergency:

NHS Direct
0845 4647
www.nhsdirect.nhs.uk
– 24-hour free medical advice

For more information about puberty and growing up:

www.wiredforhealth.gov.uk
www.teenagehealthfreak.org.uk
www.mindbodysoul.gov.uk
– lots of useful information on growing up

Sexwise
0800 28 29 30
www.ruthinking.co.uk
– free advice and information on sex and relationships for under 18s

Brook
0800 0185 023
www.brook.org.uk
– provides free, confidential contraception and sex advice for young people under 25

Family Planning Association (FPA)
◇ England & Wales   0845 310 1334
◇ Scotland   0141 576 5088
◇ N Ireland   02890 325 488
www.fpa.org.uk
– medical advice on contraception, pregnancy and STIs

If you have any problem you'd like to talk through or are depressed or having emotional difficulties, contact:

ChildLine – England, Wales, Scotland & Northern Ireland
0800 1111
www.childline.org.uk
– 24-hour free confidential helpline for young people with any problems

ChildLine – Eire (run by ISPCC)
Ireland Freephone 1800 666 666

The Line
0800 88 44 44
– ChildLine's service for young people living away from home or in care, open weekdays 3.30pm to 9.30pm, weekends 2pm to 8pm

The Samaritans
08457 90 90 90,
email: jo@samaritans.org
– 24-hour confidential helpline for young people with any problems

Anti-Bullying Campaign
020 7378 1446
www.bullying.co.uk
- advice for victims of bullying, open weekdays
10am to 4pm

Who Cares? Trust
LinkLine 0500 564 570
www.thewhocarestrust.org.uk
- support and advice for young people in care,
open Mon, Wed, Thurs 3.30pm to 6pm

Get Connected
0808 808 4994
www.getconnected.org.uk
- will find the best service to help, whatever the
problem, open 1pm to 11pm every day

No Panic
0808 808 0545
www.no-panic.co.uk
- information and support for panic attacks,
phobias, obsessive compulsive disorders (OCDs),
open 10am to 10pm every day

Cruse Bereavement Care
0870 167 1677
www.crusebereavementcare.org.uk
- advice and counselling for anyone who has been
affected by a death, open Mon, Wed, Fri
3pm to 9pm

If you have been or are being abused:

ChildLine – England, Wales, Scotland &
Northern Ireland
0800 1111
www.childline.org.uk
– 24-hour free confidential helpline for young
people with any problems

ChildLine – Eire (run by ISPCC)
Ireland Freephone 1800 666 666

NSPCC Helpline
0808 800 5000
www.nspcc.org.uk
– advice and support for any young person who has
suffered or is suffering from physical, emotional or
sexual abuse. (**NB:** This helpline does not guarantee
confidentiality in cases of serious abuse, but you
can ask for advice without disclosing your name or
location. If in doubt, check with the helpline
counsellor who will always tell you at what point
they would have to break confidentiality.)

Survivors UK
PO Box 2470, London SW9 6WQ
020 7357 6677 (Tues 7pm to 10pm only)
www.survivorsuk.org.uk
– advice and support for young men who have
been the victims of sexual abuse or male rape

Legal advice for young people:

Children's Legal Centre
01206 873820
www2.essex.ac.uk/clc
– open weekdays 10am to 12.30pm & 2pm to
4.30pm

For health information:

Acne Support Group
Howard House, The Runway,
South Ruislip, Middlesex HA4 6SE
020 8841 4747
www.stopspots.org
– advice and support for people suffering from
acne

www.wiredforhealth.gov.uk
www.mindbodysoul.gov.uk
– lots of useful information on all aspects of health
for young people

For addictions:

Alateen
020 7403 0888
www.al-anon.org/alateen.html
– advice for young people whose lives have been
affected by someone else's problem with alcohol,
open 10am to 10pm daily

Drinkline
0800 917 8282
www.healthwise.org.uk
– advice on alcohol problems, open 9am to 11pm
weekdays, 6pm to 11pm weekends

Quit
0800 002200
www.quit.org.uk
– free help and information on how to stop
smoking, open 9am to 9pm seven days a week

National Drugs Helpline
0800 776600
www.healthwise.org.uk
– 24-hour confidential advice, information and
support to anyone concerned about drug misuse

For information on HIV and AIDS:

National AIDS Helpline
0800 567 123
www.healthwise.org.uk

Terrence Higgins Trust
020 7242 1010
www.tht.org.uk
– HIV support and information

Avert
www.avert.org
– information on AIDS, sex & contraception and
homosexuality

For information about nutrition and diet while you are growing:

www.wiredforhealth.gov.uk
– lots of useful information about healthy eating and other aspects of health and growing

Eating Disorders Association
01603 621414
www.edauk.com
– support and advice for anyone experiencing difficulties with eating, open weekdays 8.30am to 8.30pm

Useful booklets and nutritional information for young people wishing to remove meat from their diet:

The Vegan Society
01424 427393
www.vegansociety.com

The Vegetarian Society
0161 925 2000
www.vegsoc.org

Addresses parents might find useful:

Family Planning Association (FPA)
FP Sales Ltd, PO Box 1078, East Oxford, Oxford
OX14 6JE
01865 719418
www.fpa.org.uk

– write or call for a free catalogue of leaflets and an excellent book list

ParentLine Plus
0808 800 2222
www.parentlineplus.org.uk
– help and information about caring for children

Trust for the Study of Adolescence
01273 693311
www.tsa.uk.com
– provides information and resources for professionals working with adolescents and parents

SANELINE
0845 767 8000
www.sane.org.uk
– advice and support for the sufferers of mental illness and their families, open 12pm to 2am daily

Glossary

Acne	Spots and red pimples on the skin. Often starts around puberty. Mainly affects the face, back and chest. Lots of treatments are available.
Addiction	State of dependence on alcohol or drugs.
Adolescence	The stage of development between childhood and adulthood.
Age of consent	The age at which a young woman can legally agree to have sex: 16 in England, Scotland and Wales, 17 in Northern Ireland. Any boy or man having sex with her before this age is breaking the law.
AIDS	Acquired Immune Deficiency Syndrome. An illness where the body is unable to fight infections due to the HIV virus.
Anaemia	Too little haemoglobin (the part of the blood which carries oxygen). Can be caused by an unhealthy diet with too little iron.
Anorexia	(Medical name: anorexia nervosa) An eating disorder where someone starves themselves because they are convinced they are overweight – despite all evidence to the contrary. Can be fatal.
Antibiotic	A type of medicine used to treat bacterial infections.

Anus	Sometimes called the back passage. The opening in your bottom where stools (poo) come out.
Areola	The darker circle of skin around the nipples.
Bacteria	Organisms (bugs) which cause infection. Often treated with antibiotics.
Balanitis	Inflammation (redness and swelling) of the penis – often associated with tightness of the foreskin.
Bisexual	An individual who is sexually attracted to men *and* women.
Blackhead	A plug formed from fatty material in the outlet of a sebaceous gland in the skin.
Bladder	A sac which stores the urine produced in the kidneys.
Breast buds	The small, sometimes tender, lumps which develop under the nipples at the start of puberty.
Breasts	Female breasts grow during puberty. They are made of milk-producing glands and fatty tissue. If a woman has a baby, they produce milk.
Bulimia	Uncontrollable overeating usually alternating with periods of undereating.
Cervix	A tight ring of muscle around the opening from a woman's uterus (womb) into her vagina. Literally means the neck of the uterus.

Circumcision | The surgical removal of the foreskin.

Clitoris | A small, very sensitive, pea-sized area in front of a woman's vagina, near where the labia minora meet.

Contraception | The prevention of pregnancy.

Cramp | A painful muscle contraction.

Cycle | A regular sequence of events. For example, a girl's menstrual cycle happens when an egg is released roughly every four weeks.

Depression | A state of feeling very sad or miserable. Can affect sleep and appetite.

Ejaculation | Sudden discharge of semen from the penis during orgasm, sometimes called 'coming'.

Erection | Enlargement and hardening of the penis – often as a result of sexual stimulation but, during puberty, frequently happens on its own.

Fallopian tubes | The two tubes between a woman's ovaries and her uterus. Eggs travel down them once a month.

Feminine hygiene products | Another name for sanitary products – pads, towels, STs, tampons. This name is often used in large shops or supermarkets.

Fertile | Able to make a woman pregnant (man) or able to become pregnant (woman).

Fertilisation	When a sperm and an egg join together.
Foetus	(Also spelled fetus.) An unborn baby which grows and develops in the uterus (womb).
Foreskin	A sleeve of skin which covers the end of the penis.
Gay	Another word for homosexual.
Genitals /genitalia	The parts of the reproductive system on the outside of the body.
Glans	The head of the penis.
Gynaecomastia	Temporary swelling of breasts in boys during puberty.
Heterosexual	Someone who is sexually attracted to the opposite sex.
Homosexual	Someone who is sexually attracted to their own sex.
Hormone	A chemical messenger, usually produced in one area of a body and acting on another area. (Important hormones for boys in puberty are growth hormone and testosterone.)
Lubrication	A slippery substance which reduces friction.
Masturbation	Touching one's own sexual parts to give pleasure.

Nipple	The part of a breast which sticks out. A baby sucks on the mother's nipple to get milk.
Oestrogen	One of the most important female hormones – causes breast growth and other changes during puberty.
Osteochondritis	Painful inflammation in an area where a tendon is attached to a bone.
Ovaries	A woman has two ovaries which produce eggs. If an egg is fertilised by a man's sperm a baby may develop. The ovaries are in the lower part of the tummy, one on either side of the uterus.
Para-phimosis	Painful condition where the foreskin is too tight to be pulled back over the erect penis.
Peer pressure	The feeling that everyone in your social or age group is doing something, so you have to do it too.
Penis	The male sexual organ. The part of a boy's or man's body that urine and sperm come out of.
Pharmacist	The person (usually wearing a white coat) in a chemist's shop (pharmacy) in charge of selling medicines and making up doctors' prescriptions. Can give lots of useful advice.
PMS	Pre-menstrual syndrome – moodiness and discomfort experienced by many girls in the days leading up to their period. Caused by changing levels of hormones.

Progesterone	An important female hormone – helps control a girl's monthly cycle of periods.
Puberty	The body changes which take place as a child develops into an adult.
Pubic	The area between the top of your legs, around your genitals, e.g., pubic hair.
Reproductive organs	The parts of the body involved in producing a baby.
Sanitary product	Products used to soak up the blood from a period. Towels, pads, STs, tampons, etc.
Scrotum	The sac (or bag) which contains a male's testes. It hangs between the legs behind the penis.
Semen	(Or seminal fluid.) The liquid containing sperm which comes out of a penis on ejaculation.
Smegma	The secretion of the glands of the foreskin.
Sperm	The male sex cells which can join with a female egg to form a baby. Sperm are made in the testes.
Stools	Another name for poo, number twos, faeces.
Straight	Another word for heterosexual.
Testicles	Another word for testes.

Testis/testes	In males there are two testes which produce sperm. Each testis is enclosed in the scrotum or bag which hangs behind the penis.
Testosterone	A male sex hormone which causes male characteristics including body hair, voice changes and development of sexual organs.
Urethra	The narrow tube that opens at the end of the penis, through which urine passes from the bladder. It also carries sperm during ejaculation.
Urine	Pee or wee. Urine is made by the kidneys and is then stored in your bladder until you go to the lavatory. Urine is made up mainly of things that your body needs to get rid of. It is usually a pale yellow colour.
Uterus	An upside down, pear shaped organ in the lower part of a woman's tummy. This is where a baby grows. It is also where blood is produced during a period.
Vagina	One of the three openings between a girl's legs. It is a muscular tube connecting the uterus and cervix to the outside.
Vas deferens	The tube which carries sperm from the testes to the penis (see diagram p. 44).
Vasectomy	An operation (usually permanent) to block the tubes that carry sperm from the testes to the penis. A form of contraception.
Womb	Another name for the uterus.

Index